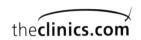
theclinics.com

OBSTETRICS AND GYNECOLOGY CLINICS OF NORTH AMERICA

Multiple Gestations

GUEST EDITORS
Isaac Blickstein, MD
Louis G. Keith, MD, PhD

March 2005 • Volume 32 • Number 1

SAUNDERS

An Imprint of Elsevier, Inc.
PHILADELPHIA   LONDON   TORONTO   MONTREAL   SYDNEY   TOKYO

W.B. SAUNDERS COMPANY
A Division of Elsevier Inc.

The Curtis Center • Independence Square West • Philadelphia, Pennsylvania 19106

http://www.theclinics.com

OBSTETRICS AND GYNECOLOGY
CLINICS OF NORTH AMERICA   Volume 32, Number 1
March 2005   ISSN 0889-8545
Editor: Carin Davis   ISBN 1-4160-2740-8

Reprints. For copies of 100 or more of articles in this publication, please contact the Commercial Reprints Department, Elsevier Inc., 360 Park Avenue South, New York, New York 10010-1710. Tel.: (212) 633-3818, Fax: (212) 462-1935, email: reprints@elsevier.com

The ideas and opinions expressed in *Obstetrics and Gynecology Clinics of North America* do not necessarily reflect those of the Publisher. The Publisher does not assume any responsibility for any injury and/or damage to persons or property arising out of or related to any use of the material contained in this periodical. The reader is advised to check the appropriate medical literature and the product information currently provided by the manufacturer of each drug to be administered to verify the dosage, the method and duration of administration, or contraindications. It is the responsibility of the treating physician or other health care professional, relying on independent experience and knowledge of the patient, to determine drug dosages and the best treatment for the patient. Mention of any product in this issue should not be construed as endorsement by the contributors, editors, or the Publisher of the product or manufacturers' claims.

Obstetrics and Gynecology Clinics of North America (ISSN 0889-8545) is published quarterly by Elsevier. Corporate and editorial offices: 170 S Independence Mall W 300 E, Philadelphia, PA 19106-3399. Accounting and circulation offices: 6277 Sea Harbor Drive, Orlando, FL 32887-4800. Periodicals postage paid at Orlando, FL 32862, and additional mailing offices. Subscription prices are $175.00 per year for US individuals, $288.00 per year for US institutions, $88.00 per year for US students and residents, $207.00 per year for Canadian individuals, $350.00 per year for Canadian institutions, $235.00 per year for international individuals, $350.00 per year for international institutions and $118.00 per year for Canadian and foreign students/residents. To receive student/resident rate, orders must be accompanied by name of affiliated institution, date of term, and the signature of program/residency coordinator on institution letterhead. Orders will be billed at individual rate until proof of status is received. Foreign air speed delivery is included in all Clinics subscription prices. All prices are subject to change without notice. POSTMASTER: Send address changes to *Obstetrics and Gynecology Clinics of North America*, W.B. Saunders Company, Periodicals Fulfillment, Orlando, FL 32887-4800. **Customer Service: 1-800-654-2452 (US). From outside of the US, call 1-407-345-4000.**

Obstetrics and Gynecology Clinics of North America is also published in Spanish by Mc Graw-Hill Interamericana Editores S.A., P.O. Box 5-237, 06500, Mexico; in Portuguese by Reichmann and Affonso Editores, Rio de Janeiro, Brazil; and in Greek by Paschalidis Medical Publications, Athens, Greece.

Obstetrics and Gynecology Clinics of North America is covered in *Index Medicus, Excerpta Medica, Current Concepts/Clinical Medicine, Science Citation Index, BIOSIS, CINAHL, and ISI/BIOMED.*

Printed in the United States of America.

GOAL STATEMENT

The goal of *Obstetrics and Gynecology Clinics of North America* is to keep practicing physicians up to date with current clinical practice in OB/GYN by providing timely articles reviewing the state of the art in patient care.

ACCREDITATION

The *Obstetrics and Gynecology Clinics of North America* is planned and implemented in accordance with the Essential Areas and Policies of the Accreditation Council for Continuing Medical Education (ACCME) through the joint sponsorship of the University of Virginia School of Medicine and W. B. Saunders Company. The University of Virginia School of Medicine is accredited by the ACCME to provide continuing medical education for physicians.

The University of Virginia School of Medicine designates this educational activity for a maximum of 60 category 1 credits per year, 15 category 1 credits per issue, toward the AMA Physician's Recognition Award. Each physician should claim only those credits that he/she actually spent in the activity.

The American Medical Association has determined that physicians not licensed in the US who participate in this CME activity are eligible for AMA PRA category 1 credit.

Category 1 credit can be earned by reading the text material, taking the CME examination online at http://www.theclinics.com/home/cme, and completing the evaluation. After taking the test, you will be required to review any and all incorrect answers. Following completion of the test and evaluation, your credit will be awarded and you may print your certificate.

FACULTY DISCLOSURE

Faculty Disclosure

As a provider accredited by the Accreditation Council for Continuing Medical Education (ACCME), the Office of Continuing Medical Education of the University of Virginia School of Medicine must ensure balance, independence, objectivity, and scientific rigor in all its individually sponsored or jointly sponsored educational activities. All authors/editors participating in a sponsored activity are expected to disclose to the readers any significant financial interest or other relationship (1) with the manufacturer(s) of any commercial product(s) and/or provider(s) of commercial services discussed in an educational presentation and (2) with any commercial supporters of the activity (significant financial interest or other relationship can include such things as grants or research support, employee, consultant, stock holder, member of speakers bureau, etc.) The intent of this disclosure is not to prevent authors/editors with a significant financial or other relationship from writing an article, but rather to provide readers with information on which they can make their own judgments. It remains for the readers to determine whether the author's/editor's interest or relationships may influence the article with regard to exposition or conclusion.

The authors/editors listed below have identified no professional or financial affiliations related to their presentation:

Greg R. Alexander, MPH, ScD; Zvi Appelman, MD; Liora Baor, PhD, MSW; Isaac Blickstein, MD; Carin Davis, Acquisitions Editor; Jan Deprest, MD, PhD; Richard P. Dickey, MD, PhD; Boris Furman, MD; Jacques Jani, MD; Louis G. Keith, MD, PhD; Russell S. Kirby, PhD, MS; Liesbeth Lewi, MD; Alexandra Matias, MD, PhD; Nuno Montenegro, MD, PhD; Jaroslaw J. Oleszczuk, MD, PhD; Agnieska K. Oleszczuk, MD; Peter O.D. Pharoah, MD, MSc; Hamisu Salihu, MD, PhD; Eric Shinwell, MD; and, Martha Slay Wingate, MPH, DrPH.

Disclosure of discussion of non-FDA approved uses for pharmaceutical products and/or medical devices: The University of Virginia School of Medicine, as an ACCME provider, requires that all authors/editors identify and disclose any "off label" uses for pharmaceutical products and/or for medical devices. The University of Virginia School of Medicine recommends that each reader fully review all the available data on new products or procedures prior to instituting them with patients.

All authors/editors who provided disclosures have indicated that they will not be discussing off-label uses.

TO ENROLL

To enroll in the *Obstetrics and Gynecology Clinics of North America* Continuing Medical Education program, call customer service at 1-800-654-2452 or visit us online at www.theclinics.com/home/cme. The CME program is available to subscribers for an additional fee of $99.95.

GUEST EDITORS

ISAAC BLICKSTEIN, MD, Professor, Department of Obstetrics and Gynecology, Kaplan Medical Center, Rehovot; Hadassah-Hebrew University School of Medicine, Jerusalem, Israel

LOUIS G. KEITH, MD, PhD, Center for Study of Multiple Birth; Feinberg School of Medicine, Northwestern University, Chicago, Illinois

CONTRIBUTORS

GREG R. ALEXANDER, MPH, ScD, Professor and Chair, Department of Maternal and Child Health, School of Public Health, University of Alabama at Birmingham, Birmingham, Alabama

ZVI APPELMAN, MD, Department of Obstetrics and Gynecology and Institute of Clinical Genetics, Kaplan Medical Center, Rehovot; Medical School of the Hebrew University and Hadassah, Jerusalem, Israel

LIORA BAOR, MSW, Faculty of Social Sciences, School of Social Work, Bar-Ilan University, Ramat-Gan, Israel

ISAAC BLICKSTEIN, MD, Professor, Department of Obstetrics and Gynecology, Kaplan Medical Center, Rehovot; Hadassah-Hebrew University School of Medicine, Jerusalem, Israel

JAN DEPREST, MD, PhD, Professor, Department of Obstetrics and Gynecology, Centre for Surgical Technologies, University Hospital Gasthuisberg, Leuven, Belgium

RICHARD P. DICKEY, MD, PhD, Chief, Section of Reproductive Endocrinology and Infertility; and Clinical Professor, Department of Obstetrics and Gynecology, Louisiana State University Medical School; Medical Director, Fertility Institute of New Orleans, New Orleans, Louisiana

BORIS FURMAN, MD, Department of Obstetrics and Gynecology, Kaplan Medical Center, Rehovot; Medical School of the Hebrew University and Hadassah, Jerusalem, Israel

JACQUES JANI, MD, Consultant, PhD Research Fellow, Department of Obstetrics and Gynecology, Centre for Surgical Technologies, Leuven, Belgium

LOUIS G. KEITH, MD, PhD, Center for Study of Multiple Birth, Feinberg School of Medicine, Northwestern University, Chicago, Illinois

RUSSELL S. KIRBY, PhD, MS, Professor, Department of Maternal and Child Health, School of Public Health, University of Alabama at Birmingham, Birmingham, Alabama

LIESBETH LEWI, MD, Consultant, PhD Research Fellow, Department of Obstetrics and Gynecology, Centre for Surgical Technologies, Leuven, Belgium

ALEXANDRA MATIAS, MD, PhD, Department of Obstetrics and Gynecology, Faculty of Medicine, Porto, University Hospital of S. João, Porto, Portugal

NUNO MONTENEGRO, MD, PhD, Department of Obstetrics and Gynecology, Faculty of Medicine, Porto, University Hospital of S. João, Porto, Portugal

AGNIESZKA K. OLESZCZUK, MD, Department of Ophthalmology, Medical Institute of the Department of Defense of the Republic of Poland, Warsaw, Poland

JAROSLAW J. OLESZCZUK, MD, PhD, McKinsey & Company; Center for Study of Multiple Birth, Chicago, Illinois

PETER O.D. PHAROAH, MD, MSc, FRCP, FRCPCH, FFPHM, Emeritus Professor, FSID Unit of Perinatal and Paediatric Epidemiology, Department of Public Health, University of Liverpool, Liverpool, United Kingdom

HAMISU SALIHU, MD, PhD, Associate Professor, Department of Maternal and Child Health, School of Public Health, University of Alabama at Birmingham, Birmingham, Alabama

ERIC S. SHINWELL, MD, Director of Neonatology, Kaplan Medical Center, Rehovot; and Senior Lecturer in Pediatrics, Hebrew University, Jerusalem, Israel

MARTHA SLAY WINGATE, MPH, DrPH, Educational Research Consultant, Department of Maternal and Child Health, School of Public Health, University of Alabama at Birmingham, Birmingham, Alabama

CONTENTS

The purpose of this article is to describe the perinatal mortality experience and mortality-related risk factors of recent US multiple births. First, we describe trends in fetal and neonatal mortality rates for singleton and multiple births to understand if the improvements in perinatal mortality in the United States are equally or differentially reflected among multiple births. Because the characteristics of women who have multiple deliveries differ from those of mothers of singletons, we describe the risk of fetal and neonatal mortality by maternal characteristics and plurality. Finally, we examine the distribution and fetal and neonatal mortality risk of singleton and multiple births by birth weight and gestational age to provide an updated assessment and contrast of their comparative survival chances within similar birth weight–gestational age categories of intrauterine development.

Spontaneous reduction of multiple gestational sacs occurs less often in pregnancies conceived as a result of ovulation induction and assisted reproductive technology compared with spontaneously conceived multiple pregnancies. Whereas most spontaneous multiple pregnancies are twin gestations, a higher proportion of multiple pregnancies that result from ovulation induction and assisted reproductive technology are triplet and higher-order gestations. Recent evidence, described in this article, indicates that although twin and higher-order multiple gestations found on initial ultrasound subsequently may undergo spontaneous reduction to singletons or twins, there may be important consequences for the outcome of the surviving fetus or fetuses.

The epidemic of multiple births has translated into a marked rise in very low birth weight infants, who are at risk for major neonatal morbidity and mortality. Gestational age–adjusted comparisons of outcome betweens singletons and multiples have shown conflicting results. Comparisons that corrected for relevant confounding variables show that twins and singletons have similar risks for early morbidity and mortality. Very low birth weight triplets may have increased risk for neonatal mortality, however. Second-born very low birth weight twins seem to be at risk for increased respiratory morbidity, even in the era of routine antenatal corticosteroids and postnatal surfactant therapy.

Growth of twins and higher-order multiples is an exceptional metabolic challenge for the expecting mother. She is doing much more than a mother of a singleton in terms of nurturing, however. Metabolic requirements need adequate dietary intervention in the form of increased weight gain during early pregnancy. It is normal for multiples to be smaller than singletons. Being smaller than singletons does not necessarily mean that multiples are pathologically growth restricted. It is important to remember that twins and triplets have different growth patterns, and their growth should not be considered by using singleton standards. When a small-for-gestational-age fetus is suspected in a multiple pregnancy, it is advisable to follow or to treat the pregnancy as if it was an SGA singleton.

Multiple compared with singleton gestations have a five- to ten-fold increased risk of CP. The increased risk associated with MC placentation has been variously ascribed to transfer of thromboplastin or thromboemboli from the dead to the surviving fetus, exsanguination of the surviving fetus into the low pressure reservoir of the dead fetus, or hemodynamic instability with bidirectional shunting of blood between the two fetuses. An increased risk of CP in assisted reproductive technology gestations is to be expected because of the higher proportion of preterm births. The increase in risk of CP associated with monochorionic placentation will not be observed except for the minority of assisted reproductive technology gestations that undergo monozygotic splitting.

FORTHCOMING ISSUES

RECENT ISSUES

The Clinics are now available online!
http://www.theclinics.com

ELSEVIER
SAUNDERS

Obstet Gynecol Clin N Am
32 (2005) xiii–xiv

OBSTETRICS AND
GYNECOLOGY
CLINICS
OF NORTH AMERICA

Preface

Multiple Gestations

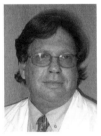 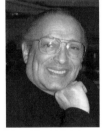

Isaac Blickstein, MD   Louis G. Keith, MD, PhD
Guest Editors

As recently as the early 1980s, twin pregnancy and birth was a relatively rare event, and higher-order multiples were of negligible consequence. However, this did not deter clinicians as well as researchers from evaluating the clinical management of multiples. Obviously, the validity of many of these studies was hampered because of small sample size and underpowered statistics. Beginning in the early 1980s, all we knew about the natural history of multiples has been profoundly changed. Physician-made (iatrogenic) multiple pregnancies are now seen in most developed countries with frequencies approaching 50% in twins and more than 75% in higher-order multiples. The resultant demographic trends—and now a serious public health issue—may be summarized in two major points:

- First, the frequency of twins has almost doubled, and that of higher-order multiples has increased 400% to 600%. These changes translate immediately into a greater and significant proportion of multiples among premature and low–birth weight infants. Preterm birth and growth aberrations are indeed the most important adverse consequences of the so-called "epidemic" of multiple gestations.
- Second, whereas in the past mothers had their last child in their late 30s, at present these mothers are giving birth to their firstborn. This trend, associated with a greater need for assisted conceptions, disproportionately

0889-8545/05/$ – see front matter © 2005 Elsevier Inc. All rights reserved.
doi:10.1016/j.ogc.2004.11.001

obgyn.theclinics.com

increases the number of mothers of multiples among elderly parturients. Inevitably, those mothers are in greater need for invasive and noninvasive diagnostic measures to exclude aneuploidy.

In this issue of the *Obstetrics and Gynecology Clinics of North America*, we first present a series of papers discussing the perinatal mortality risks of multiples, embryonic loss following assisted conceptions, neonatal morbidity, and growth aberrations. These perinatal considerations are followed by a discussion of the increased risk of long-term morbidity – cerebral palsy. To complement the epidemiologic and clinical data, the paradox of older maternal age in multiples is discussed. We then present the problems associated with genetic diagnosis and the use of sophisticated antenatal interventions to diagnose and treat complicated cases. Finally, we wish to understand why—despite the above-mentioned potential complications—infertile women still prefer that their infertility treatment result in multiple births.

We wish to thank all of the authors for their scholarly contributions to this issue. We also thank Ms. Carin Davis, our Editor, for her continuous help and support.

Isaac Blickstein, MD
Obstetrics & Gynecology
Kaplan Medical Center
76100 Rehovot, Israel
E-mail address: blick@netvision.net.il

Louis G. Keith, MD, PhD
Feinberg School of Medicine
Northwestern University
333 E. Superior, Room 464
Chicago, IL 60611, USA
E-mail address: lgk395@northwestern.edu

ELSEVIER
SAUNDERS

Obstet Gynecol Clin N Am
32 (2005) 1–16

OBSTETRICS AND
GYNECOLOGY
CLINICS
OF NORTH AMERICA

Fetal and Neonatal Mortality Risks of Multiple Births

Greg R. Alexander, MPH, ScD*,
Martha Slay Wingate, MPH, DrPH, Hamisu Salihu, MD, PhD,
Russell S. Kirby, PhD, MS

*Department of Maternal and Child Health, School of Public Health,
University of Alabama at Birmingham, RPHB 320, 1530 3rd Avenue South,
Birmingham, AL 35294-0022, USA*

Over the past two decades, perinatal mortality in the United States has declined substantially. From 1980 to 2001, the rate of infant mortality (death of a live birth up to 1 year after birth) declined 46%, from 12.6 to 6.8 infant deaths per 1000 live births [1]. Neonatal mortality (death of a live birth between 0 and 27 days after birth) declined from 8.5 neonatal deaths per 1000 live births in 1980 to 4.5 in 2001, a 47% decrease. Fetal mortality (20 or more weeks' gestation) dropped from 9.1 fetal deaths per 1000 live births plus fetal deaths in 1980 to 6.5 in 2001, a relatively less marked but still notable decrease of 29%. These improvements in perinatal survival seem to be largely caused by decreasing risks of gestational age and birth weight–specific mortality [2–4], which reflect technologic and medical advances in high-risk obstetric and neonatal care and diagnostics, including ultrasound, antenatal steroids, high-frequency ventilation, and exogenous surfactant [5–17]. Regionalization of perinatal services and efforts to increase earlier entry into prenatal care have organized and facilitated access and timely use of these perinatal services among high-risk populations [18–20].

Although these advances in perinatal care and improvements in perinatal survival are laudable, many challenges still face the perinatal field. During the past two decades, low birth weight (ie, <2500 g) and preterm (<37 weeks' gestation) birth rates have increased steadily [21]. This situation has drawn the

This work was supported in part by DHHS, HRSA, MCHB grant 6T76MC00008.

* Corresponding author.

E-mail address: alexandg@uab.edu (G.R. Alexander).

obgyn.theclinics.com

attention of researchers and policy analysts, who seek to better delineate the various factors behind the swelling proportion of infants born too small and too soon and understand our evident failure to reverse the continual rise in numbers. One often cited contributor to these trends in the United States and elsewhere is the dramatic increase over the last 20 years in the rate and number of multiple births [22]. Multiple births have higher rates of infant mortality and are at a greatly increased risk of low birth weight and preterm delivery [23,24]. According to previous research, at least 50% of all twins and 90% of all triplets and higher-order multiples are low birth weight or preterm [25]. The number of twins in the United States rose 65% from 68,339 in 1980 to 125,134 in 2002. Between 1980 and 1998, the rate of higher-order multiples increased from 37 to 193.5 per 100,000 live births. Although twin rates continue to climb, the explosive rise in triplets and higher-order multiples (eg, quadruplets, quintuplets) seen in the 1980s and 1990s has subsided, at least temporarily. In 2002, there were 6898 triplets, 434 quadruplets, and 69 quintuplets and other higher-order births in the United States, and the rate of triplet and other higher-order multiples per 100,000 was down 1% from 2001 [22].

Several factors have been suggested for this rising incidence in multiple births in the United States. Frequently proposed as a primary determinant of this trend is the development and use of assisted reproductive technologies (ART) [24,26,27]. The dramatic increase in triplets, quadruplets, and higher-order multiples stemming from ART has led obstetric and gynecologic organizations to call for the reduction in multiple birth deliveries associated with ART [28–30], because infants who are products of higher-order multiple births are at substantial increased risk for adverse outcomes, such as ventricular hemorrhages, cerebral palsy, and other conditions that potentially lead to disabilities in later life [31].

In conjunction with the rising use of ART has been a shift in the age demographics of the US maternity population. The average age of a mother at time of delivery has risen markedly in the United States over the past two decades. Increases in the rates of multiple births, particularly twins and triplets, in most developed nations also can be contributed to the rising maternal age observed. Older mothers have an increased likelihood of spontaneous multiple births; there is also an increasing association of multiple births with advancing maternal age, because the necessity for using ART increases as a result of the accumulation of conditions that predispose to infertility [24–26]. Previous studies estimate that between one fourth and one third of the increase in the twin and triplet rates can be attributed solely to the increase in maternal ages without the impact of fertility treatments [23].

The purpose of this article is to describe the perinatal mortality experience and mortality-related risk factors of recent US multiple births. First, we describe trends in fetal and neonatal mortality rates for singleton and multiple births to understand if the improvements in perinatal mortality in the United States are equally or differentially reflected among multiple births. With this information, we can assess better the impact of the rise in multiple births on perinatal mortality trends. Because the characteristics of women who have multiple deliveries differ from the mothers of singletons, we describe the risk of fetal and neonatal mortality by maternal characteristics and plurality to offer a clearer understanding of the extent to which the association of traditional maternal risk factors with fetal and neonatal mortality varies among singleton and multiple births. Finally, we examine the distribution and fetal and neonatal mortality risk of singleton and multiple births by birth weight and gestational age to provide an updated assessment and contrast of their comparative survival chances within similar birth weight–gestational age categories of intrauterine development. For these analyses, we draw on databases from the US National Center of Health Statistics, including the 1985 to 1988 and 1995 to 1998 Linked Live Birth/Infant Death Cohort Files and the Fetal Death files from the US Perinatal Mortality Data File and the 1995 to 1998 Matched Multiple Linked Files [32–40].

Trends in fetal and neonatal mortality

Table 1 examines temporal changes in fetal and neonatal mortality by plurality (singletons, twins and triplets, and higher-order multiples). Using the 1985 to 1988 and 1995 to 1998 US Live Birth/Infant Death Linked Cohort and Fetal Death files, we calculated fetal and neonatal mortality rates from the two time periods. For fetal death, we considered early (20–27 weeks' gestation), late ($\geq$28 weeks' gestation), and overall fetal mortality rates per 1000 live births and fetal death deliveries. For neonatal and perinatal mortality rates, the denominators were live births in the given time period. We then calculated the percent change from the period during 1985 to 1988 to the period during 1995 to 1998 for each plurality group.

Although substantial decreases in perinatal mortality rates among singletons over the last decade occurred, even more marked declines are evident for twins and triplets and higher-order multiples. Between 1985 and 1988 and 1995 and 1998, the perinatal mortality rate for singletons declined from 12.76 to 10.45, a nearly 18% decrease. Over the same period, the decline in perinatal mortality for twins was nearly 30% and for triplets and higher-order multiples was more than 40%. Similar patterns are evident for neonatal and fetal mortality, with the greatest improvement in mortality rates being observed for the higher-order multiples. For early fetal mortality (20–27 weeks' gestation), singletons experienced an increase in mortality risk in contrast to declining early fetal mortality rates for multiple births. The potential influence of temporal variation in accuracy and completeness of fetal death reporting for singletons and multiples must be considered when interpreting this increase.

Although there has been a greater improvement in perinatal mortality among multiples compared with singletons, an appreciable disparity by plurality in the risk of fetal and neonatal mortality remains. Compared with singleton births, in 1995 to 1998, twins still had approximately four times the risk of perinatal mortality, and higher-order multiple births had perinatal mortality rates that were nearly nine times higher. There are morbidities associated with the multiple

Table 1
Fetal and neonatal mortality rates by plurality 1985 to 1988 and 1995 to 1998 fetal death and live born deliveries to US resident mothers

	Early fetal mortality rate[a] (per 1000 deliveries)			Late fetal mortality rate[b] (per 1000 deliveries)			Fetal mortality rate[c] (per 1000 deliveries)			Neonatal mortality rate[d] (per 1000 live births)			Perinatal mortality rate[e] (per 1000 deliveries)		
	1985–1988	1995–1998	% Change	1985–1988	1995–1998	% Change	1985–1988	1995–1998	% Change	1985–1988	1995–1998	% Change	1985–1988	1995–1998	% Change
Singletons	2.55	2.92	14.51	4.62	3.53	−23.59	7.17	6.45	−10.18	5.54	4.01	−27.62	12.67	10.45	−17.52
Twins	12.73	12.30	−3.38	13.01	7.65	−41.20	25.74	19.95	−22.49	39.32	25.66	−34.74	64.05	45.10	−29.59
Triplets or higher-order multiples[f]	22.05	19.15	−13.15	16.31	9.11	−44.14	38.37	28.26	−26.35	114.79	62.24	−45.78	148.75	88.74	−40.34

[a] Early fetal mortality rate: fetal deaths 20–27 weeks' gestation per 1000 deliveries (live birth plus fetal deaths).
[b] Late fetal mortality rate: fetal deaths ≥28 weeks' gestation per 1000 deliveries (live birth plus fetal deaths).
[c] Fetal mortality rate: fetal deaths ≥20 weeks' gestation per 1000 deliveries (live birth plus fetal deaths).
[d] Neonatal mortality rate: deaths occurring 0–27 days after live birth per 1000 live births.
[e] Perinatal mortality rate: fetal deaths ≥20 weeks' gestation and deaths occurring 0–27 days after live birth per 1000 deliveries (live birth plus fetal deaths).
[f] Quadruplets and higher-order multiples cannot be separated from triplets because of reporting on 1985–1988 fetal death and live birth certificates.
Data from US National Center for Health Statistics: Linked live birth/infant death cohort files, 1985–1988 and 1995–1998; US Fetal Death files, 1995–1998. Hyattsville (MD): Public Health Service.

deliveries that survive. Given that the United States continues to rank poorly among developed nations in infant mortality rates and has dropped comparatively lower in its standing in the last several decades, the recent decline in overall US perinatal mortality rates may have been even more profound had it not been for the markedly increasing proportion of US births that are multiple births.

Fetal mortality by maternal characteristics

Maternal demographics

Table 2 provides unadjusted fetal mortality rates by selected maternal characteristics and plurality. Using the 1995 to 1998 US Linked Live Birth/Infant Death Cohort files, the fetal death files from the US Perinatal Mortality Data Files, and the US Matched Multiple Linked files, we calculated overall fetal mortality rates for each plurality group. For each maternal or other descriptive characteristic, we calculated the mortality rate for each plurality group. For smoking, we excluded cases with missing data and used information only from women who reported whether they smoked.

The fetal mortality rates are presented per 1000 deliveries (ie, live births plus fetal deaths) and range from 6.44 for singletons to 37.99 for quadruplets. A

Table 2
1995–1998 fetal mortality rates by maternal characteristics and plurality

	Singletons	Twins	Triplets	Quadruplets
Total fetal mortality rate	6.44	20.02	26.80	37.99
Demographics and maternal characteristics				
Non-Hispanic whites	4.92	16.78	20.67	34.43
Non-Hispanic blacks	10.87	24.86	54.28	—
Hispanics	5.58	19.27	36.84	—
Other/unknown race	12.75	45.29	72.21	—
Unmarried	12.84	41.00	126.6	217.82
Teen (<20 y)	8.05	34.55	88.71	—
Average age (20–34 y)	5.85	19.54	27.95	43.42
Older age (≥35 y)	8.42	16.20	20.36	20.62
High education (13+ y)	4.48	15.27	21.87	36.57
Male	6.72	20.66	29.61	40.70
Female	6.15	19.38	23.97	35.20
Primigravida	5.88	26.81	35.39	68.70
High gravidity for age[a]	12.97	22.12	33.49	41.20
Previous pregnancy loss	31.13	72.62	111.46	239.44
Tobacco use	7.79	20.29	54.72	—

[a] High gravidity for age is defined as having equal to or more than the following number of previous deliveries: 2+ for mothers <18 years, 3+ for mothers 18–21 years, 4+ for mothers 22–24 years, 5+ for mothers 25–29 years, and 6+ for mothers 30+ years.
Data from US linked live birth/infant death cohort files, 1995–1998 for singletons; US matched multiple linked, 1995-1998; US fetal death files, 1995–1998. Hyattsville (MD): Public Health Service.

generally increasing risk of fetal mortality by plurality was apparent for every maternal characteristics subgroup. Within each plurality group, non-Hispanic whites had the lowest unadjusted fetal mortality rates, whereas the other/ unknown race group had the highest rates. Fetal mortality rates among non-Hispanic black singletons and triplets were more than double that of non-Hispanic whites—a white-black disparity consistently observed in many adverse birth outcomes indicators [4,41]. Across plurality groups, fetal unadjusted mortality rates that were consistently higher than average also were evident for the following criteria: unmarried teen (<20 years of age), high gravidity for age, previous pregnancy loss, and tobacco use. Although singleton deliveries to older women (35 or more years of age) demonstrated higher fetal mortality rates, multiple gestations to older women evinced lower-than-average risks of fetal death.

Adjusted odds ratios for maternal characteristics

For selected maternal characteristics, Table 3 presents adjusted odds ratios for the risk of fetal death for singletons, twins, and triplets. Using the live birth/infant death, fetal death, and multiples files, we calculated the odds ratios and 95% confidence intervals for each plurality group, controlling for race, marital status, age, education, parity, sex, previous pregnancy loss, and smoking. For singletons, significantly higher fetal mortality risks were found for male sex deliveries and for deliveries to women with the following characteristics: black race, other/ unknown race, unmarried, age 35 or older, and previous pregnancy loss. Compared with the white reference group, twin deliveries to Hispanic and non-Hispanic black mothers were found to have a significantly lower risk of fetal death. For twins and triplets, single marital status, previous pregnancy loss, primigravida, male sex, and other/unknown race were found to contribute to

Table 3
Adjusted odds ratios for the risk of fetal mortality by singleton and multiple births

	Singletons	Twins	Triplets
Non-Hispanic blacks	1.14 (1.12–1.16)	0.73 (0.69–0.77)	0.76 (0.58–0.99)
Hispanics	0.82 (0.80–0.84)	0.78 (0.73–0.84)	1.00 (0.74–1.35)
Other/unknown race	2.41 (2.36–2.45)	2.39 (2.23–2.57)	3.52 (2.68–4.61)
Unmarried	4.09 (4.03–4.16)	4.01 (3.88–4.31)	10.88 (8.88–13.32)
Teen (<20 y)	0.78 (0.77–0.80)	0.92 (0.85–0.99)	0.90 (0.60–1.34)
Older (≥35 y)	1.69 (1.66–1.72)	0.97 (0.91–1.04)	0.79 (0.64–0.97)
High education (13+ y)	0.75 (0.74–0.76)	0.83 (0.70–0.87)	1.03 (0.84–1.25)
Male	1.10 (1.08–1.11)	1.07 (1.03–1.12)	1.21 (1.02–1.43)
Primigravida	0.95 (0.94–0.97)	1.57 (1.49–1.66)	1.91 (1.55–2.36)
High gravidity for age	0.64 (0.63–0.66)	0.40 (0.36–0.44)	0.30 (0.21–0.41)
Previous pregnancy loss	5.88 (5.74–6.02)	7.65 (7.06–8.29)	10.87 (8.40–14.07)
Tobacco use	0.82 (0.81–0.84)	0.67 (0.62–0.72)	1.11 (0.77–1.61)

Reference group: Non-Hispanic white, married, average age (20–34 years), ≤12 years education, average parity-for-age, female, no previous pregnancy loss, no tobacco use reported.
Data from US linked live birth/infant death cohort files, 1995–1998 for singletons; US matched multiple linked, 1995–1998; US fetal death files, 1995–1998. Hyattsville (MD): Public Health Service.

significantly higher odds of experiencing a fetal death, whereas for twins, the deliveries of mothers characterized as being younger than 20 years, having high education, and using tobacco had lower-than-average risks of fetal death. Although increased maternal age ($\geq$35 years) was a significant risk factor for fetal death for singleton births, for triplets it entailed a lower risk of fetal death comparable to that of average aged mothers (20–34 years). High gravidity for age was a highly protective factor for all plurality groups.

Neonatal mortality by maternal characteristics

Maternal demographics

Table 4 provides unadjusted neonatal mortality rates by selected maternal characteristics and plurality. Using the 1995 to 1998 US Linked Live Birth/Infant Death Cohort files, the fetal death files from the US Perinatal Mortality Data Files, and the US Matched Multiple Linked files, we first calculated overall unadjusted neonatal mortality rates. For each demographic subgroup, we calculated the unadjusted mortality rate for each plurality group.

Neonatal rate for singletons is approximately 4 neonatal deaths per 1000 live births, and the rate dramatically rises with increasing number at birth to a rate of more than 67 for quadruplets. The disparities in neonatal mortality rates between blacks and whites are evident among multiples and singletons. Hispanics, non-

Table 4

1995–1998 neonatal mortality rates by maternal characteristics and plurality

	Singletons	Twins	Triplets	Quadruplets
Total neonatal mortality	4.01	23.65	53.73	67.54
Demographics and maternal characteristics				
Non-Hispanic whites	3.23	20.70	49.36	66.13
Non-Hispanic blacks	8.13	38.78	94.08	—
Hispanics	3.41	22.31	75.88	89.82
Other/unknown race	3.83	24.14	64.04	—
Unmarried	5.74	32.91	86.79	—
Teen (<20 y)	5.47	46.28	144.54	—
Average age (20–34 y)	3.72	23.84	60.57	82.11
Older ($\geq$35 y)	4.41	16.68	37.03	31.60
High education (13+ y)	3.01	19.50	47.02	69.70
Male	4.40	26.24	58.92	56.89
Female	3.65	22.02	51.50	83.83
Primigravida	4.00	29.37	57.66	57.38
High gravidity	7.02	26.28	60.51	58.59
Previous pregnancy loss	8.69	34.21	62.28	92.59
Tobacco use	5.23	27.32	98.41	—

Data from US linked live birth/infant death cohort files, 1995–1998 for singletons; US matched multiple linked, 1995–1998. Hyattsville (MD): Public Health Service.

Hispanic whites, and other/unknown race groups had roughly similar neonatal mortality rates for singletons and twins, greater differences were evident for triplets. For all plurality groups, neonatal mortality rates are higher for infants of mothers with the following characteristics: black race, other/unknown race, unmarried status, age younger than 20 years, tobacco use, and previous pregnancy losses.

Adjusted odds ratios for maternal characteristics

Table 5 provides adjusted odds ratios for neonatal death for selected maternal characteristics. As with fetal mortality odds ratios, using the live birth/infant death, fetal death, and multiples files, we calculated the odds ratios and 95% confidence intervals for each plurality group, controlling for race, marital status, age, education, parity, sex, previous pregnancy loss, and smoking. For singletons, significantly higher neonatal mortality risks were found for deliveries with the following characteristics: black race, other/unknown race, unmarried, younger than age 20 or age 35 or older, male gender, primigravida or high gravidity for age, previous pregnancy loss, and tobacco use. High education and Hispanic ethnicity were the only maternal factors with a significantly lower risk of neonatal mortality for singletons. For twin deliveries, Hispanics were found to have a risk of neonatal mortality nearly similar to whites. For triplets, the Hispanic risk of neonatal death was significantly greater than whites. Twins and triplets who were male or were born to teen (<20 years) mothers were found have significantly higher odds of experiencing a neonatal death. Maternal age of 35 or more years was a significant risk factor for neonatal death in singletons but was a protective characteristic for twins and triplets.

Table 5
Adjusted odds ratios for the risk of neonatal mortality by singleton and multiple births

	Singletons	Twins	Triplets
Non-Hispanic blacks	2.13 (2.08–2.17)	1.61 (1.536–1.70)	1.65 (1.33–2.04)
Hispanics	0.95 (0.93–0.97)	0.94 (0.88–1.01)	1.34 (1.06–1.78)
Other/unknown race	1.19 (1.15–1.23)	1.16 (1.06–1.27)	1.37 (1.06–1.78)
Unmarried	1.26 (1.24–1.29)	1.10 (1.04–1.15)	0.98 (0.80–1.21)
Teen (<20 y)	1.06 (1.03–1.09)	1.53 (1.4–1.63)	1.76 (1.25–2.48)
Older (≥35 y)	1.27 (1.24–1.30)	0.76 (0.71–0.81)	0.62 (0.54–0.72)
High education (13+ y)	0.72 (0.71–0.73)	0.80 (0.76–0.83)	0.72 (0.63–0.82)
Male	1.21 (1.19–1.24)	1.20 (1.15–1.25)	1.16 (1.03–1.30)
Primigravida	1.05 (1.03–1.07)	1.28 (1.22–1.35)	1.09 (0.93–1.27)
High gravidity for age	1.17 (1.13–1.21)	0.94 (0.86–1.02)	0.93 (0.74–1.19)
Previous pregnancy loss	1.85 (1.77–1.92)	1.65 (1.49–1.84)	1.27 (0.95–1.69)
Tobacco use	1.19 (1.16–1.22)	1.06 (0.99–1.13)	1.69 (1.29–2.22)

Reference group: Non-Hispanic white, married, average age (20–34 years), ≤12 years education, average parity-for-age, female, no previous pregnancy loss, no tobacco use reported.
Data from US linked live birth/infant death cohort files, 1995–1998 for singletons; US matched multiple linked, 1995–1998. Hyattsville (MD): Public Health Service.

Birth weight and gestational age–specific proportion and rates

For each plurality group, singletons to quadruplets, Table 6 presents the proportion of deliveries, fetal deaths, and neonatal deaths for birth weight–gestational age categories. Using the 1995 to 1998 US Linked Live Birth/Infant Death Cohort files, the fetal death files from the US Perinatal Mortality Data Files, and the US Matched Multiple Linked files, proportions of total deliveries, fetal deaths, and neonatal deaths were calculated. The birth weight categories were classified into six groups: (1) less than 500 g, (2) 500 to 749 g, (3) 750 to 1499 g, (4) 1500 to 2499 g, (5) 2500 to 3999 g, and (6) 4000 to 8500 g. Gestational age categories were categorized into five groups: (1) less than 28 weeks, (2) 28 to 32 weeks, (3) 33 to 36 weeks, (4) 37 to 41 weeks, and (5) more than 42 weeks' gestation. The percent of total deliveries included all live births and fetal deaths from 1995 to 1998.

The first section of Table 6 shows the total deliveries, that is, the percent of live births plus fetal deaths by birth weight–gestational age category with separate birth weight and gestational age summary totals. For singletons, most (>80%) deliveries occurred between 37 and 41 weeks' gestation and 2500 to 3999 g. Most twin deliveries were found from 37 to 41 weeks' gestation and 1500 to 3999 g. For triplets, the highest proportion of deliveries was between 33 and 36 weeks' gestation at birth weights 1500 to 2499 g. For quadruplets, nearly 50% or more of deliveries were 28 to 32 weeks' gestation and 750 to 1499 g. Whereas more than 10% of triplets and quadruplet deliveries were less than 28 weeks' gestation, less than 1% of singletons and only 5% of twins were delivered extremely preterm.

The second part of Table 6 displays by plurality groups the percent of fetal deaths distributed by birth weight and gestational age categories. More than 60% of fetal deaths of multiple deliveries but 45% of fetal deaths of singleton deliveries occur at gestational ages less than 28 weeks' gestation. More than 20% of singleton fetal deaths are at term or later, whereas most fetal deaths to multiples occur at lower birth weights and gestational ages.

For each plurality group, the third section of Table 6 presents the percentage of neonatal death distributed by birth weight–gestational age categories. Regardless of plurality, most neonatal deaths occur among infants delivered before 28 weeks' gestation and at birth weights less than 1500 g. Nearly 90% of neonatal deaths to quadruplets occur to infants delivered before 28 weeks' gestation. Reflecting the scarcity of higher-order multiple births at normal birth weight or at term, a scant proportion of neonatal deaths of multiple births occur at the higher birth weight and gestational age categories. For singletons, however, more than 20% of neonatal deaths occur at birth weights between 2500 and 3999 g and at gestational ages 37 to 41 weeks.

Birth weight and gestational age–specific fetal and neonatal mortality rates are provided in Table 7 for each plurality group. Fetal mortality rates are in the first section. These rates were reported per 1000 deliveries. Birth weight and gestational age categories are identical to Table 6. For deliveries at less than

Table 6

Percent of deliveries for birth weight and gestational age categories by plurality: 1995–1998 deliveries to US residents

BW/Gest	<28				28–32				33–36				37–41				42+				Total			
Plurality	S	Tw	Trip	Quad	S	Tw	Trip	Quad	S	Tw	Trip	Quad	S	Tw	Trip	Quad	S	Tw	Trip	Quad	S	Tw	Trip	Quad
Percent of live births plus fetal deaths																								
4000–8500					0.3	0.4	0.2		0.2				9.1	0.2		0.2	1.1	1.0	0.1	0.1	10.4	0.2	0.0	0.3
2500–3999		0.1			0.6	5.5	15.0	17.5	5.5	13.2	4.9	0.5	71.3	31.1	1.7	0.4	6.1	0.5	0.3	0.1	83.2	45.6	6.9	1.0
1500–2499			0.2		0.5	4.3	17.4	34.7	2.2	24.9	38.5	17.1	2.1	12.1	4.2	1.1	0.1	0.0	0.1	0.2	5.0	43.1	58.1	35.9
750–1499	0.3	1.9	4.7	8.6		0.3	0.7	1.7	0.1	1.1	3.7	5.7	0.0	0.2	0.5	0.6	0.0				0.9	7.5	26.5	49.6
500–749	0.3	1.7	4.3	6.5							0.1										0.3	2.0	5.0	8.2
<500	0.2	1.5	3.5	4.9																	0.2	1.5	3.5	4.9
Total	0.8	5.2	12.7	20.0	1.4	10.5	33.3	53.8	8.0	39.2	47.2	23.3	82.5	43.6	6.4	2.3	7.4	1.5	0.5	0.4	100.0	99.9	100.0	99.9
Percent of fetal deaths																								
4000–8500					0.4	0.2			0.2				1.8	0.1			0.3	0.1			2.2	0.1		
2500–3999		0.2			4.1	3.3	2.4		4.2	2.0	0.9		14.6	2.9	0.9		1.2	0.1			20.4	5.2	1.8	
1500–2499	0.3				7.6	8.6	9.3	18.8	8.1	7.9	4.0		4.8	3.9	1.1		0.3	0.3			17.6	15.6	7.5	
750–1499	5.4	5.7	3.3	1.6	2.4	2.7	5.5	6.3	2.9	3.6	5.3	4.7	0.7	0.9	0.2		0.1	0.1			16.6	18.9	18.1	25.1
500–749	13.0	14.1	10.8	9.4	1.1	1.7	2.4	1.6	0.2	0.2	0.2										15.5	17.0	16.5	15.7
<500	26.5	41.6	53.5	54.7																	27.6	41.6	55.9	56.3
Total	45.2	61.6	67.6	65.7	15.6	16.5	19.6	26.7	15.4	13.7	10.4	4.7	21.8	7.8	2.3	0.0	1.9	0.5			99.9	98.4	99.9	97.1
Percent of neonatal deaths																								
4000–8500					0.4	0.1							1.5				0.2				1.8			
2500–3999		0.1			3.1	1.9	0.9		3.5	0.9	0.1		16.5	1.7	0.1		1.7				22.0	2.7	0.3	
1500–2499	0.3		0.2		5.2	6.7	6.2	4.0	5.6	3.9	2.0		4.7	1.7	0.2		0.4	0.1			14.1	7.8	3.2	
750–1499	7.5	9.4	7.8	9.5	1.6	2.6	1.4	2.4	1.4	1.7	1.1	0.8	0.5	0.3							14.7	18.1	15.1	14.3
500–749	22.8	32.6	35.4	36.5	0.7	1.1	0.3	1.6		0.2											24.4	35.4	36.8	38.9
<500	22.1	34.8	44.2	43.7																	22.8	34.8	44.5	45.2
Total	52.7	76.9	87.6	89.7	11.0	12.5	8.8	7.9	10.5	6.8	3.2	1.6	23.2	3.7	0.3		2.3	0.1			99.8	98.8	99.9	98.4

Total cells may not add up to 100% because of small number of births at specific birth weight–gestational age category.

Abbreviations: BW/Gest, birth weight/gestational age; Quad, quadruplet; S, singleton; Trip, triplet; Tw, twin.

Table 7
Fetal and neonatal mortality rates for birth weight and gestational age categories by plurality: 1995–1998 deliveries to US residents

BW/Gest	<28				28–32				33–36				37–41				42+				Total			
Plurality	S	Tw	Trip	Quad	S	Tw	Trip	Quad	S	Tw	Trip	Quad	S	Tw	Trip	Quad	S	Tw	Trip	Quad	S	Tw	Trip	Quad
Fetal mortality rates[a]																								
4000–8500									4.8				1.1	10.1			1.2				1.2	10.2		
2500–3999					8.4	8.8			4.1	2.5	3.6		1.1	1.5	10.4		1.1	1.1	1.0		1.3	1.9	6.9	
1500–2499	90.27	32.9			37.5	9.5	3.2		20.2	5.1	2.1		12.1	5.1	5.2		14.1	10.2			18.9	5.9	2.8	
750–1499	115.4	48.9	14.0	5.7	92.1	32.2	10.6	16.9	138.7	51.4	27.3	25.9	99.8	67.5	9.3		79.9	40.0			105.5	41.8	13.8	15.8
500–749	275.7	130.0	50.6	45.1	316.7	158.9	163.4		701.0												283.2	142.9	71.2	59.5
<500	597.8	431.9	306.8	346.5	591.8	406.0															597.5	457.1	354.7	354.0
Total	318.1	187.8	107.5	102.2	62.3	25.0	11.9	16.2	10.6	5.6	4.3	8.4	1.4	2.8	6.9		1.4	4.7						
Neonatal mortality rates[b]																								
4000–8500									2.6				0.6	6.7			0.7				0.7	7.3		
2500–3999					5.5	8.1			2.4	1.6	0.9		0.9	1.2			1.0				1.0	1.3	1.9	
1500–2499	47.65	24.6			19.7	7.8	3.0		9.6	3.5	2.6		8.2	3.2	2.6		11.7	1.0			10.4	4.0	2.8	
750–1499	109.3	113.0	83.1	68.2	43.3	34.7	18.0	2.8	46.8	33.2	15.4	2.9	56.2	33.2	2.1		34.3	4.4			64.0	53.6	29.0	2.7
500–749	332.9	418.4	419.0	345.9	147.8	218.9	104.6	7.1	46.4												306.5	391.3	372.5	17.7
<500	341.4	502.1	640.2	544.6	234.3	383.5															336.9	515.7	641.5	291.7
Total	254.0	326.1	350.3	274.9	30.1	26.5	13.4	9.9	5.0	3.8	3.5	4.2	1.0	1.9	2.1		1.2	2.0	9.3					

Total cells may not add up to 100% because of small number of births at specific birth weight–gestational age category.
[a] Fetal mortality rates: per 1000 deliveries.
[b] Neonatal mortality rates: per 1000 live births.

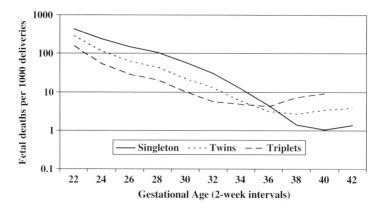

Fig. 1. Gestational age-specific fetal mortality by plurality, 1995 to 1998.

37 weeks' gestation or less than 2500 g, singleton births exhibit the highest fetal mortality rates. In these birth weight–gestational age categories, twins have the next higher fetal mortality rate. For 2-week intervals, Fig. 1 presents gestational age–specific fetal mortality rates for singletons, twins, and triplets. This graph more clearly displays the variations in mortality risk by plurality and reveals that only at term is there a survival advantage for singletons births compared with multiples. Fig. 2 provides an alternative approach to presenting these data and presents the risk of fetal mortality using a denominator of fetuses at risk. The prospective risk of fetal mortality was calculated as a proportion of the total number of fetuses at risk at a given gestational age. The number of fetuses at risk was calculated by consecutive subtraction of weekly deliveries (ie, live births),

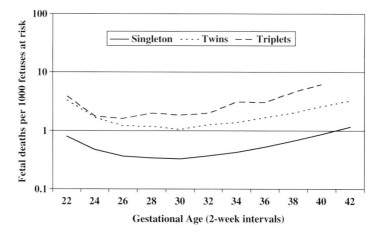

Fig. 2. Gestational age-specific prospective risk of fetal mortality by plurality, 1995 to 1998.

fetal deaths, or otherwise. This number differs from the fetal death rate because it is calculated as a proportion of total deliveries at a given gestational age [42]. Although multiples have a lower gestational age–specific mortality at earlier gestational age, their higher proportion of extremely preterm births results in an elevated risk of mortality for undelivered fetuses at risk across the entire gestational age range.

The second section of Table 7 provides birth weight–gestational age–specific neonatal mortality rates by plurality. Rates were calculated similarly to fetal death rates, but the denominator consisted of only live births. At the earliest gestational age and lightest birth weight category, singletons have preferential neonatal mortality rates. Between 28 and 32 weeks' gestation and 500 to 2500 g, however, neonatal mortality rates are lower for each increasingly higher order of multiple births. At term and normal birth weight deliveries, singletons demonstrate the lowest risk of neonatal death.

Summary

The risk of fetal and neonatal death for twins, triplets, and higher-order multiple births declined markedly over the last decade. The decline in perinatal mortality risk among multiple gestations is even greater than that observed for singletons. Although delineating the various precursors that may underlie this observed improvement in survival is beyond the scope of this article, these findings suggest that ongoing advances have been made in the clinical management of multiple births. These advances have lessened the potential impact that the growing increase in multiple gestations might have had on the total population's perinatal health indicators. Pregnancies with multiple deliveries entail heightened risks of fetal and infant mortality and subsequent morbidity for survivors. The birth weight–gestational age mortality curves of singletons are inappropriate for establishing the mortality risk of multiple deliveries at specific birth weights and gestational ages. Although on average increasingly higher-order multiple births are delivered earlier and smaller, at these gestational age and birth weight categories they exhibit better survival than singletons. The survival advantage of higher-order multiple erodes with increasing gestational age, and their mortality risk appreciably exceeds that of singletons at term and normal birth weights.

The results of this analysis have clinical and public health implications. The maternal characteristics identified in this analysis (eg, black race, age, education, marital status, previous pregnancy loss) are generally well known and established. What may be less well understood, however, is that whereas some of the risk markers elevate the susceptibility of the fetus to an adverse pregnancy event (eg, fetal demise) among singletons, they are protective among multiples. For instance, advanced maternal age ($\geq$35 years) heightens the risk for fetal and neonatal mortality among singletons, whereas among multiples, infants of older mothers fare better than infants of their younger counterparts. This information could be critical in classifying patients according to risk and prognostic criteria based on which appropriate interventions are targeted. Still, many classically used maternal sociodemographic risk characteristics for singleton births are applicable for multiple births (eg, black race of mother). Not only do some of these indicators differ in terms of their relationship with fetal versus neonatal mortality (eg, for singleton births, high gravidity for age is a high risk factor for neonatal mortality but is a protective low risk factor for fetal mortality) but also they differ for singleton versus multiple deliveries (eg, for triplets, Hispanic mothers are at increased risk of neonatal death but not fetal death).

Beyond the clinical implications of the findings, the complex interrelationship of sociodemographic characteristics with the risk of multiple birth and the risk of subsequent perinatal mortality highlights the intricate sociocultural dynamic underpinning the increasing multiple birth trend. To the extent that higher perinatal mortality rates presage equally elevated risks of morbidity, developmental delay, and the need for long-term care, the relatively greater risks of adverse outcomes of multiple births are of consequence for policy makers and public health practitioners who strive to ensure the availability of needed follow-up services to families while containing health care costs. Despite improvements in the survival of multiple births, the increase in their incidence is a serious matter for concern, which likely will continue to fuel debates about policies related to ART.

References

[1] Centers for Disease Control and Prevention. Infant mortality and low birth weight among black and white infants: United States, 1980–2000. MMWR Morb Mortal Wkly Rep 2002;51:589–92.
[2] Lee KS, Paneth N, Gartner LM, et al. Neonatal mortality: an analysis of the recent improvement in the United States. Am J Public Health 1980;70(1):15–21.
[3] Allen MC, Alexander GR, Tompkins ME, et al. Racial differences in temporal changes in newborn viability and survival by gestational age. Paediatr Perinat Epidemiol 2000;14:152–8.
[4] Alexander GR, Tompkins ME, Allen MC, et al. Trends and racial differences in birth weight and related survival. Matern Child Health J 1999;3(1):71–9.
[5] Goldenberg RL, Rouse DJ. Prevention of premature birth. N Engl J Med 1998;339(5):313–20.
[6] Goldenberg RL. The prevention of low birth weight and its sequela. Prev Med 1994;23:627–31.
[7] Ballard PL. Scientific rationale for the use of antenatal glucocorticoids to promote fetal development. Pediatr Rev 2000;1(5):E83–90.
[8] Thorp JM, Hartmann KE, Berkman ND, et al. Antibiotic therapy for the treatment of preterm labor: a review of the evidence. Am J Obstet Gynecol 2002;186:587–92.
[9] Curley AE, Halliday HL. The present status of exogenous surfactant for the newborn. Early Hum Dev 2001;61(2):67–83.
[10] Eichenwald EC, Stark AR. High-frequency ventilation: current status. Pediatr Rev 1999;20(12): e127–33.
[11] Horbar JD, Lucey JF. Evaluation of neonatal intensive care technologies. Future Child 1995;5(1): 139–61.
[12] Reger R, Dolfin T, Ben-Nun Y, et al. Survival rate and 2-year outcome in very low birth weight infants. Isr J Med Sci 1995;31(5):309–13.
[13] Schwartz RM, Luby AM, Scanlon JW, et al. Effects of surfactant on morbidity, mortality, and resource use in newborn infants weighing 500 to 1500 g. N Engl J Med 1994;330(21):1476–80.

[14] Avery ME, Tooley WH, Keller JB, et al. Is chronic lung disease in low birth weight infants preventable? A survey of eight centers. Pediatrics 1987;79(1):26–30.

[15] Copper RL, Goldenberg RL, Creasy RK, et al. A multicenter study of preterm birth weight and gestational age-specific neonatal mortality. Am J Obstet Gynecol 1993;168(1):78–84.

[16] Howell EM, Vert P. Neonatal intensive care and birth weight-specific perinatal mortality in Michigan and Lorraine. Pediatrics 1993;91(2):464–70.

[17] Philip AGS. Neonatal mortality rate: is further improvement possible? J Pediatr 1995;126(3): 427–32.

[18] Hulsey TC, Heins HC, Marshall TA, et al. Regionalized perinatal care in South Carolina. J S C Med Assoc 1989;85(8):357–84.

[19] Alexander GR, Kogan MD, Nabukera S. Racial differences in prenatal care use in the United States: are the disparities decreasing? Am J Public Health 2002;92(12):1970–5.

[20] Kogan MD, Martin J, Alexander GR, et al. The changing pattern of prenatal care utilization in the US, 1981–1995: using different prenatal care indices. JAMA 1998;279(20):1623–8.

[21] Arias E, MacDorman MF, Strobino DM, et al. Annual summary of vital statistics: 2002. Pediatrics 2003;112(6):1215–30.

[22] Martin JA, Hamilton BE, Venture SJ, et al. Births: final data for 2001. National vital statistics reports; vol. 51. no. 2. Hyattsville (MD): National Center for Health Statistics; 2002.

[23] Blondel B, Kaminski M. Trends in the occurrence, determinants, and consequences of multiple births. Semin Perinatol 2002;26(4):239–49.

[24] Reynolds MA, Shieve LA, Martin JA, et al. Trends in multiple births conceived using assisted reproductive technology, United States, 1997–2000. Pediatrics 2003;111(5, Part 2):1159–62.

[25] Russell RB, Petrini JR, Damus K, et al. The changing epidemiology of multiple births in the United States. Obstet Gynecol 2003;101(1):129–35.

[26] Jewell SE, Yip R. Increasing trends in plural births in the United States. Obstet Gynecol 1995;85: 229–32.

[27] Misra DP, Ananth CV. Infant mortality among singletons and twins in the United States during 2 decades: effects of maternal age. Pediatrics 2002;110(6):1163–8.

[28] Templeton A. Avoiding multiple pregnancies in ART: replace as many embryos as you like, one at a time. Hum Reprod 2000;15:1662.

[29] Olivennes F. Double trouble: yes a twin pregnancy is an adverse outcome. Hum Reprod 2000;15: 1663–5.

[30] Campus Course Report ESHRE. Prevention of twin pregnancies after IVF/ICSI by single embryo transfer. Hum Reprod 2001;16:790–800.

[31] Polin JI, Frangipane WL. Current concepts in management of obstetric problems for pediatricians. II. Modern concepts in the management of multiple gestations. Pediatr Clin North Am 1986;33:649–61.

[32] National Center for Health Statistics. Matched multiple birth data set: 1995–1998. CD-ROM Series 21, No. 13a. Hyattsville (MD): Public Health Service; 2003.

[33] National Center for Health Statistics. 1998 birth cohort linked birth/infant death data set. CD-ROM Series 20, No. 16a. Hyattsville (MD): Public Health Service; 2002.

[34] National Center for Health Statistics. 1997 birth cohort linked birth/infant death data set. CD-ROM Series 20, No. 15a. Hyattsville (MD): Public Health Service; 2002.

[35] National Center for Health Statistics. 1996 birth cohort linked birth/infant death data set. CD-ROM Series 20, No. 14a. Hyattsville (MD): Public Health Service; 2002.

[36] National Center for Health Statistics. 1995 birth cohort linked birth/infant death data set. CD-ROM Series 20, No. 12a. Hyattsville (MD): Public Health Service; 2002.

[37] National Center for Health Statistics. 1998 perinatal mortality data file. Series 20, No. 18. Hyattsville (MD): Public Health Service; 2000.

[38] National Center for Health Statistics. 1997 perinatal mortality data file. Series 20, No. 15. Hyattsville (MD): Public Health Service; 1999.

[39] National Center for Health Statistics. 1996 perinatal mortality data file. Series 20, No. 14. Hyattsville (MD): Public Health Service; 1998.

ALEXANDER et al

[40] National Center for Health Statistics. 1995 perinatal mortality data file. Series 20, No. 12. Hyattsville (MD): Public Health Service; 1998.

[41] Kessel SS, Kleinman JC, Koontz AM, et al. Racial differences in pregnancy outcomes. Clin Perinatol 1988;15(4):745–54.

[42] Kahn B, Lumey LH, Zybert PA, et al. Prospective risk of fetal death in singleton, twin and triplet gestations: implications for practice. Obstet Gynecol 2003;102(4):685–92.

ELSEVIER
SAUNDERS

Obstet Gynecol Clin N Am
32 (2005) 17–27

OBSTETRICS AND
GYNECOLOGY
CLINICS
OF NORTH AMERICA

Embryonic Loss in Iatrogenic Multiples

Richard P. Dickey, MD, PhD[a,b],*

[a]*Fertility Institute of New Orleans, 6020 Bullard Avenue, New Orleans, LA 70128, USA*
[b]*Section of Reproductive Endocrinology and Infertility, Department of Obstetrics and Gynecology,*
Louisiana State University Medical School, 1542 Tulane Avenue, New Orleans, LA 70112, USA

Multiple conceptions are a frequent consequence of ovulation induction (OI) and in vitro fertilization (IVF), gamete intrafallopian transfer (GIFT), or related assisted reproductive technologies (ART). In 2000, 118,997 babies were born as twins and 7328 were born as triplets, quadruplets, and higher orders in the United States [1]. Of this number, OI without ART was estimated to be responsible for 20% of twin births and 38% of triplet and higher-order multiple births; ART produced 11% of twin births and 45% of higher-order multiple births; spontaneous conceptions accounted for 69% of twins and 17% of higher-order multiple births [2]. The number of multiple births would be even higher if it were not for selective reduction, spontaneous reduction, or early gestational sacs (GS) or embryonic loss of one or more concepti.

The occurrence of spontaneous reduction in multiple pregnancies is perhaps most noticeable in iatrogenic pregnancies after infertility treatment because pelvic ultrasound (US) is usually performed earlier than in spontaneous pregnancies to confirm the presence of an intrauterine gestation. In a comprehensive review of the literature before 1995 concerning early fetal loss in multiple gestations, Landy and Nies [3] found 35 reports that comprised 1542 multiple gestations, predominantly twins, diagnosed by US. Most twins occurred spontaneously, and in most of these cases the first US was performed after the ninth week of gestation. In one study of 126 twin pregnancies in which US was performed earlier in some cases, the subsequent loss rate of one sac was 29% when the first US was performed before 7 weeks' gestation compared with a subsequent loss rate of 17% when the first US was performed from 7 to 9 weeks' gestation [4]. In a 1990

---

* Fertility Institute of New Orleans, 6020 Bullard Avenue, New Orleans, LA 70128.
E-mail address: info@fertilityinstitute.com

study of 274 multiple pregnancies by the present author, the probability of a twin birth after two embryonic heart rates were present 7 weeks' gestation or later was 90% for maternal age younger than 30 years and 84% for age 30 or older [5]. By contrast, when two GS were present on an initial US performed during weeks 5 to 6, the probability of a twin birth was 63% for age younger than 30 years and 52% for age 30 or older. In the studies reviewed by Landy and Nies [3], loss of one or more concepti in multiple pregnancies ranged in frequency from 10.5% to 100%. Differences in the gestational age at the time the first US was performed and in maternal age account for much of these differences in the observed rate of spontaneous absorption reported in the past. Another cause of this disparity may be whether pregnancies were the result of OI or ART [5,6].

The rate of occurrence of spontaneous loss in multiple implantations that do not progress to a size that can be distinguished on US after OI and ART can never be known but may be much higher than the rate observed after early US. There is a nine- to tenfold range in quantitative human chorionic gonadotropin serum concentrations 14 to 15 days after ART procedures in pregnancies with single GS 21 days later that subsequently deliver normal babies [7]. This finding suggests that many multiple implantations are reabsorbed before they can be recognized. As is shown in this article, multiple implantations—although they are subsequently reabsorbed—have important consequences for the outcome of the surviving fetus or fetuses.

In infertility practices, the diagnosis of multiple gestation is usually made at 5.5 to 6 weeks when a US is performed to confirm an intrauterine pregnancy. Multifetal reduction procedures are usually performed between 11 and 13 weeks. Patients and clinicians often feel the need to make decisions about management of triplet and higher-order multiple gestation pregnancy 5 to 8 weeks before Multifetal pregnancy reduction (MFPR) can be performed. An important element in this decision is whether the multiple pregnancy will undergo spontaneous reduction. The remainder of this article reviews the incidence of spontaneous reduction of GS and embryos in iatrogenic pregnancies that result from OI and ART and compares these incidences to the incidence in spontaneous pregnancy. It also examines the effect that additional implantations early in pregnancy may have on the surviving fetus or fetuses. It is primarily based on retrospective studies performed using the Fertility Institute of New Orleans' database, which contains nearly complete first-trimester and outcome data on more than 8000 pregnancies [6].

The Fertility Institute of New Orleans' experience

Between July 1, 1976 and August 31, 2000, pregnancies occurred in 8071 patients as a result of infertility treatment in our clinic. Data on all pregnancies were entered in a computer database when a pregnancy was initially confirmed by rising quantitative beta human chorionic gonadotropin levels and were updated throughout the first trimester and after delivery as additional information was obtained. Collected information included maternal age and reproductive history, infertility treatment, including type and dose of fertility drugs (if any), date of conception or last menstrual period, the number of GS and embryos present, and the date of delivery, birth weight, and type of delivery. A US was performed to determine the location and number of GS when quantitative beta human chorionic gonadotropin levels were expected to be 2000 mIU/mL or more between 5.5 and 6.5 gestational weeks (3.5–4.5 weeks after ovulation). US was repeated every 2 weeks until 12 weeks' gestation, after which time patients who continued with singleton and twin pregnancies were referred to their own obstetrician for the remainder of prenatal care and delivery. Patients with continuing triplet and higher-order multiple pregnancies were referred to a maternal fetal medicine specialist for consultation regarding MFPR, prenatal care, and delivery. The birth outcomes of 95% of singleton and twin pregnancies and of all triplet and higher-order continuing pregnancies were known through follow-up reports from patients or their obstetricians.

Multiple GS were diagnosed on initial US in 726 pregnancies (561 twin, 137 triplet, 27 quadruplet, 5 quintuplet, and 1 sextuplet). A single intrauterine GS was present in 6184 pregnancies. Excluded from subsequent analysis were 2 monochromic twin pregnancies and 35 singleton, 9 twin, 4 triplet, and 2 quadruplet pregnancies that resulted from oocyte or embryo donation because of possible disparity between the ages of the birth mother and the donor. Excluded from birth outcome analysis were 3 twin, 1 triplet, and 2 quadruplet pregnancies in which elective termination was performed and 1183 singleton, 51 twin, 7 triplet, and 1 quadruplet pregnancies that ended in first-trimester abortion. Also excluded from outcome analysis were 5 triplet, 4 quadruplet, 2 quintuplet, and 1 sextuplet pregnancies in which MFPR was performed and 305 singleton and 23 twin pregnancies in which delivery outcome was unknown.

Type of infertility treatment

The frequency of spontaneous loss of one or more GS between the initial US performed between 5 and 6 weeks' gestation and 12 weeks' gestation according to type of infertility treatment is shown in Table 1. On average, 69% of pregnancies that began as twins were continuing as viable twins at 12 weeks after clomiphene citrate, human menopausal gonadotropin (hMG)/follicle-stimulating hormone (FSH) without ART, or IVF/GIFT. By comparison, only 38% of twins conceived without fertility treatment were continuing at 12 weeks. The difference was highly significant ($P < 0.001$) and was not the result of maternal age. The frequency of loss per GS in twin pregnancies was 43% for spontaneous pregnancy, 19% after clomiphene citrate, 23% after hMG/FSH without ART, and 21% after IVF/GIFT. By comparison, spontaneous loss (abortion) occurred before the 12 weeks' gestation in 19% of singleton pregnancies conceived spontaneously or after clomiphene citrate and in 21% of singleton pregnancies conceived after hMG/FSH either with or without ART.

Table 1
Effect of ovulation induction drugs on multiple pregnancies continuing at twelve weeks

Treatment	Patients	Number fetuses continuing					Loss rate[c]
2 sacs	**Number**	**Age**	**0 (%)**	**1 (%)**	**2 (%)**		
None	56	31.0	13 (23.2)	22 (39.3)	21 (37.5)[b]		0.43
Clomiphene	211	29.8	15 (7.1)	50 (23.7)	146 (69.2)		0.19
hMG/FSH[a]	122	30.9	11 (9.0)	35 (28.7)	76 (62.3)		0.23
IVF/GIFT	160	31.8	14 (8.8)	39 (24.4)	107 (66.9)		0.21
3 sacs	**Number**	**Age**	**0 (%)**	**1 (%)**	**2 (%)**	**3 (%)**	
None	5	29.6	2 (40.0)	2 (40.0)	0 (0.0)	1 (10.0)	0.67
Clomiphene	24	31.1	1 (4.2)	4 (16.7)	14 (58.3)	5 (20.8)	0.35
hMG/FSH[a]	30	31.3	3 (10.0)	3 (10.0)	13 (43.3)	11 (36.7)	0.31
IVF/GIFT	73	32.0	1 (1.4)	4 (5.5)	21 (28.8)	47 (64.4)	0.15
4 sacs	**Number**	**Age**	**0 (%)**	**1 (%)**	**2 (%)**	**3 (%)**	**4 (%)**
None	0	—	0 (0.0)	0 (0.0)	0 (0.0)	0 (0.0)	0 (0.0)	—
Clomiphene	2	28.0	0 (0.0)	0 (0.0)	2 (100.0)	0(0.0)	0 (0.0)	0.50
hMG/FSH[a]	7	30.0	0 (0.0)	0 (0.0)	2 (28.6)	2 (28.6)	3 (42.8)	0.22
IVF/GIFT	14	32.5	1 (7.1)	0 (0.0)	4 (28.6)	4 (28.6)	5 (35.7)	0.29

[a] Not IVF or GIFT.

[b] None versus clomiphene citrate, $P < 0.0001$. None versus hMG/FSH, $P < 0.01$. None versus IVF/GIFT, $P < 0.001$.

[c] Initial number of GS: number of embryos continuing at 12 weeks divided by initial number of GS.

Adapted from Dickey RP, Taylor SN, Lu PY, et al. Spontaneous reduction of multiple pregnancy: incidence and effect on outcome. Am J Obstet Gynecol 2002;186:77–83; with permission.

Similar results were for pregnancies that began as triplets and quadruplets, although the numbers were too small to reach statistical significance. In contrast to the effect of clomiphene citrate on continuation of twin pregnancies, which was not different from hMG/FSH and IVF/GIFT, only 21% of triplet pregnancies conceived after clomiphene citrate were continuing at 12 weeks compared with 37% for hMG/FSH and 64% for IVF. When pregnancies began as quadruplet implantations after hMG/FSH and IVF/GIFT, 43% and 36%, respectively, were continuing as quadruplets and 29% were continuing as triplets at 12 weeks.

Maternal age

The effect of age on outcome of multiple pregnancies without regard to type of treatment is shown in Table 2. The probability that a GS in a multiple pregnancy would be spontaneously reabsorbed was related to the initial number of GS ($r = 0.27$, $P < 0.001$) and to maternal age ($r = 0.12$, $P < 0.01$). For twins, there was little effect of age on spontaneous loss until age 40 and older. The percent of

Table 2
Effect of maternal age on multiple pregnancies continuing at twelve weeks

Age (y)	Patients (n)	Number fetuses continuing					Loss rate[a]
2 sacs		**0 (%)**	**1 (%)**	**2 (%)**			
< 30	235	18 (7.7)	60 (25.5)	157 (66.8)			0.20
30–34	196	20 (10.2)	53 (27.0)	123 (62.8)			0.24
35–39	105	10 (9.5)	29 (27.6)	66 (62.8)			0.23
≥ 40	13	3 (23.1)	5 (38.5)	5 (38.5)			0.42
Total	549	51 (9.3)	147 (26.8)	351 (63.9)			0.23
3 sacs		**0 (%)**	**1 (%)**	**2 (%)**	**3 (%)**		
< 30	43	2 (4.6)	6 (14.0)	12 (27.9)	23 (53.5)		0.23
30–34	58	2 (3.4)	5 (8.6)	23 (39.7)	28 (48.3)		0.22
35–39	28	4 (14.3)	3 (10.7)	11 (39.3)	10 (35.7)		0.35
≥ 40	3	0 (0.0)	0 (0.0)	2 (66.7)	1 (33.3)		0.22
Total	132	8 (6.1)	14 (10.6)	48 (36.4)	62 (47.0)		0.25
4 sacs		**0 (%)**	**1 (%)**	**2 (%)**	**3 (%)**	**4 (%)**	
< 30	8	0 (0.0)	0 (0.0)	4 (50.0)	1 (12.5)	3 (37.5)	0.28
34–35	11	0 (0.0)	0 (0.0)	3 (27.3)	4 (36.4)	4 (36.4)	0.23
35–39	4	1 (25.0)	0 (0.0)	1 (50.0)	1 (25.0)	1 (25.0)	0.42
≥ 40	0	0 (0.0)	0 (0.0)	0 (0.0)	0 (0.0)	0 (0.0)	0.00
Total	23	1 (4.3)	0 (0.0)	8 (34.8)	6 (26.1)	8 (34.8)	0.28

[a] Initial number of GS: number of embryos continuing at 12 weeks divided by initial number of GS.

Adapted from Dickey RP, Taylor SN, Lu PY, et al. Spontaneous reduction of multiple pregnancy: incidence and effect on outcome. Am J Obstet Gynecol 2002;186:77–83; with permission.

twins that continued as twins at 12 weeks' gestation was 69% for age younger than 30 years, 63% for ages 30 to 34 and 35 to 39, and 38% for age 40 or older. The percent of triplet gestations that continued as triplets at 12 weeks was 54% for age younger than 30 years, 48% for ages 30 to 34, 36% for ages 35 to 39, and 33% for age 40 or older. The percent of quadruplets that continued at 12 weeks was 38% for age younger than 30, 36% for ages 30 to 34, and 25% for ages 35 to 39.

Effect of number of initial gestational sacs on length of pregnancy

The effect of the initial number of GS seen by US on the length of gestation in pregnancies that spontaneously reduced to singleton and twin pregnancies before term is shown in Tables 3 and 4. The length of gestation regardless of type of infertility treatment in pregnancies that continued past 24 weeks' gestation was inversely related to the initial number of GS for single and twin births (see Table 3). After spontaneous reduction, the average length of gestation for singleton births was shortened by 10 days when there were three GS initially

Table 3
Length of gestation by birth number and gestational sac number on initial ultrasound

Length of Gestation[a]				< 24		25–28		29–32		33–36		37–40		> 40	
	#	Days	Weeks	#	%	#	%	#	%	#	%	#	%	#	%
Singleton															
1 GS	4683	275 ± 17	39.3	148	3.2	15	0.3	41	1.0	183	3.9	2155	46.0	2141	45.7
2 GS	140	272 ± 17[b]	38.9	0	0.0	0	0.0	2	1.4	14	10.0	75	53.6	49	35.0
3 GS	14	265 ± 33[c]	37.9	0	0.0	1	7.1	1	7.1	0	0.0	7	50.0	5	35.7
Twins															
2 GS	336	254 ± 21	36.3	13	3.9	11	3.3	19	5.7	92	27.4	178	53.0	23	6.8
3 GS	48	250 ± 19[d]	35.7	0	0.0	1	2.1	3	6.2	18	37.5	24	50.0	2	4.2
4 GS	8	243 ± 17[e]	34.7	1	12.5	0	0.0	2	25.0	3	38.5	2	25.0	0	0.0
Triplets															
3 GS	57	230 ± 25	32.9	2	3.5	10	17.5	8	14.0	25	43.8	12	21.0	0	0.0
4 GS	6	225 ± 20	32.1	0	0.0	0	0.0	2	33.3	4	66.7	0	0.0	0	0.0
Quadruplets															
4 GS	4	223 ± 3	31.9	1	25.0	0	0.0	2	50.0	1	25.5	0	0.0	0	0.0
5 GS	1	—	—	1	100.0	0	0.0	0	0.0	0	0.0	0	0.0	0	0.0
Quintuplets															
5 GS	2	215	30.7	1	50.0	0	0.0	1	50.0	0	0.0	0	0.0	0	0.0

[a] Length gestation mean ± standard deviation for pregnancies delivered after completion of the twenty-fourth week.
[b] Different from one GS, P < 0.05.
[c] Different from one GS, P < 0.01.
[d] Different from two GS, P < 0.01.
[e] Different from two GS, P < 0.001.

Adapted from Dickey RP, Taylor SN, Lu PY, et al. Spontaneous reduction of multiple pregnancy: incidence and effect on outcome. Am J Obstet Gynecol 2002;186:77–83; with permission.

Table 4
Length of gestation by number of initial gestational sacs

Births Treatment No. sacs	No.	Length Gestation[a] (d)	Preterm (d)	24–32 wk		<37 wk[b]		≥37 wk	
				No.	%	No.	%	No.	%
Single birth									
None									
1 GS	2680	276.6	−3.4	34	1.3	126	4.7	2554	95.3
IVF/ART									
1 GS	261	274.8	−5.2	3	1.1	19	7.3	242	93.7
2 GS	41	271.6	−8.4	1	2.4	5	12.2	36	87.8
≥3 GS	5	264.1	−15.8	0	—	1	20.0	4	80.0
Twin birth									
None									
2 GS	21	254.5	−25.5	2	9.5	8	38.1	13	61.9
IVF/ART									
2 GS	106	251.8	−28.2	11	10.4	44	41.5	62	58.5
3 GS	21	248.3	−31.7	3	14.3	10	47.6	11	52.4
≥4 GS	4	236.5	−43.5	1	25.0	3	75.0	1	25.0

[a] From adjusted onset of menstruation; assumes ovulation or oocytes retrieval day 14.

[b] < 37 wk = 24.0 to 36.6 weeks inclusive.

Adapted from Dickey RP, Sartor BM, Pyrzak R. No single outcome measure is satisfactory when evaluating success in assisted reproduction: both twin births and singleton briths should be counted as successes. Hum Reprod 2004;19:783–7; with permission.

($P < 0.01$) and by 3 days when there were two GS initially ($P < 0.05$) compared with singleton pregnancies that began as singleton gestations. The average length of twin births was shortened by 11 days to 243 days (34.7 weeks) ($P < 0.001$) when there were four GS initially and by 4 days to 250 days (35.7 weeks) ($P < 0.01$) when there were three GS initially compared with an average length of gestation for unreduced twin pregnancies of 254 days (36.6 weeks). In general, these differences were reflected in the percent of pregnancies delivered before 37 weeks' gestation.

Additional analysis, restricted to only IVF/GIFT pregnancies presented in Table 4, shows that 15% of singleton births and 19% of twin births after IVF began as higher-order gestations [8]. Singleton births after IVF that began as single, twin, and triplet or higher-order gestations were born 1.8 days, 5 days, and 12.4 days earlier, respectively, compared with spontaneous singleton births that began as single gestations. Twin births as a result of IVF that began as twin, triplet, and quadruplet or higher-order GS were born 2.7 days, 6.2 days, and 18 days earlier, respectively, compared with spontaneous twin births that began as twin gestations. In the absence of spontaneous reduction from higher-order gestations, the proportion of singletons and twins as a result of IVF born before 32 weeks' gestation was not increased compared with spontaneously conceived singletons and twins. This information, which was not presented before 2004, indicates that the increased incidence of premature birth reported for IVF singleton and twin births compared with spontaneous pregnancies may be caused largely by the initial occurrence of triplet and higher-order gestations.

Effect of number of initial gestational sacs on weight at birth

The effect of the initial number of GS seen by US on birth weight in pregnancies that spontaneously reduced to singleton and twin pregnancies before term, regardless of type of infertility treatment, is shown in Table 5. There was a trend toward decreased birth weight as the number of initial GS increased for spontaneously reduced pregnancies, compared with unreduced pregnancies with singleton births ($r = -0.05$, $P = 0.002$) and twin births ($r = -0.15$, $P = 0.003$) (Table 5). Restricted fetal growth (intrauterine growth restriction) was defined as a birth weight less then the tenth percentile for gestational age on the basis of national singleton birth weights [9]. The incidence of restricted fetal growth for gestational age in infants from singleton births was lower than in infants from twin ($P < 0.001$) and triplet ($P < 0.05$) births. There was no consistent relationship between the incidence of restricted fetal growth and the initial number of GS in pregnancies that spontaneously reduced to a lower birth number.

Table 5
Birth weight and intrauterine growth retardation by birth number and number of gestational sacs

| Birth number | Initial Number of Gestational Sacs | | | |
	1	2	3	4
Singleton				
Patient no.	4683	140	14	0
Average weight (g)	3360 ± 599	3200 ± 650[b]	3132 ± 879[b]	—
RFG (IUGR)/infant[a]	4.5%	15.7%	14.3%	—
Twins				
Patient no.		336	48	8
Average weight (g)		2453 ± 575	2334 ± 577[c]	2024 ± 668[c]
RFG (IUGR)/infant		14.1%	11.4%	6.2%
One with RFG		17.3%	16.7%	12.5%
Two with RFG		5.3%	6.2%	0
Triplets				
Patient no.			57	6
Average weight (g)			1816 ± 598	1541 ± 276
RFG (IUGR)/infant			7.0%	11.1%
One with RFG			19.3%	33.3%
Two with RFG			1.8%	0
Three with RFG			0	0

[a] Percent babies < tenth percentile for gestational age.
[b] $P = 0.002$.
[c] $P = 0.003$.

Adapted from Dickey RP, Taylor SN, Lu PY, et al. Spontaneous reduction of multiple pregnancy: incidence and effect on outcome. Am J Obstet Gynecol 2002;186:77–83; with permission.

Comment

The principal finding of these studies, which was not appreciated previously, is that multiple pregnancies that undergo spontaneous reduction, especially from three or more initial GS to a lower number, deliver earlier and have lower birth weights than unreduced pregnancies with the same birth number. In cases of spontaneous reduction to singleton births, the differences may be too small to be clinically significant; however, twin births were more likely to occur before 36 weeks' gestation after spontaneous reduction from three or four GS.

A second important finding is that the incidence of spontaneous reduction in multiple pregnancies conceived as a result of OI and ART is no greater and seems to be less than in noniatrogenic multiple pregnancies. The reasons for this are not known but may be caused by the generally higher progesterone levels and increased uterine blood flow that result from OI. A second reason could be that leading follicles in OI, and embryos in ART, are more likely to be of the same size, which obviates the effect that earlier ovulation or larger embryo might have on later ovulation or a smaller embryo competing for the same intrauterine site.

Although it is generally accepted that after MFPR of quadruplet and higher-order pregnancies the remaining twins deliver earlier and are of lower birth weight than unreduced twins [10–16], it is less certain that this also occurs after MFPR of triplets to twins. Ours was the first study to show that the average length of gestation and weight of twins, which had spontaneously reduced from quadruplets and triplets, was less than unreduced twins conceived in our clinic. The average length of gestation and weight of singleton births that had spontaneously reduced from triplets and twins was less than unreduced singleton pregnancies conceived in our clinic. The differences in average birth weight were small and probably not clinically important: 119 g (4 oz) when twins spontaneously reduced to singleton births or triplets spontaneously reduced to twin births. The differences were larger and potentially clinically important, however—228 to 429 g (8–15 oz)—when triplets were spontaneously reduced to singletons or quadruplets were spontaneously reduced to twin or triplet births.

The incidence of restricted fetal growth (intrauterine growth restriction) after spontaneous reduction was less than half that reported by Depp et al [15] after MFPR to twins, although we used the same standard for the tenth percentile of normal singleton weight as they did [9]. In agreement with other studies [17,18], we did not find an increase in restricted fetal growth with increasing numbers of initial GS that Depp et al [15] reported. Depp et al [15], however, were the first to suggest that the differences in outcome between twins that resulted from MFPR and unreduced twins were not the result of the MFPR procedure, as had been suggested by others [13,14,19]. Instead, they proposed that first-trimester "crowding" of the developing gestations or lack of appropriate sites for placental implantation may be determining factors in placental expansion and ultimate fetal growth. Our findings support the hypothesis that impairment of early placental development because of multiple implantation sites is the cause of early delivery after MFPR and spontaneous reduction. The fact that the percent of embryos that continue at 12 weeks' gestation was related to the number of initial GS ($r = 0.31$) signifies that placental crowding is also a factor in spontaneous reduction of multiple pregnancies before 12 weeks.

The findings of these studies show that spontaneous reduction is a common occurrence in multiple pregnancies, and they suggest that the decision to perform MFPR does not need to be finalized until the mid to latter part of the first trimester. Obstetricians who manage iatrogenic multiple pregnancies in which there are initially three or more GS, although they later are reduced spontaneously to singletons or twins, should be aware that such pregnancies may deliver 4 to 10 days earlier, with babies weighing 119 g (4 oz) to 429 g (15 oz) less than unreduced singletons and twins.

References

[1] Martin JA, Hamilton BE, Vemtura SJ, et al. Births: final data for 2000. Vital Health Stat 2002; 50:1–101.

[2] Reynolds MA, Schieve LA, Martin JA, et al. Trends in multiple births conceived using assisted reproductive technology, United States, 1997–2000. Pediatrics 2003;111:1159–62.

[3] Landy HJ, Nies BM. The vanishing twin. In: Keith LG, Papiernik E, Keith DM, et al, editors. Multiple pregnancy: epidemiology, gestation and perinatal outcome. London: Parthenon Publishing Group; 1995. p. 59–71.

[4] Sampson A, de Crespigny LC. Vanishing twins: the frequency of spontaneous fetal reduction of a twin pregnancy. Ultrasound Obstet Gynecol 1992;2:107–12.

[5] Dickey RP, Olar TT, Curole DN, et al. The probability of multiple births when multiple gestational sacs or viable embryos are diagnosed at first trimester ultrasound. Hum Reprod 1990; 5:880–2.

[6] Dickey RP, Taylor SN, Lu PY, et al. Spontaneous reduction of multiple pregnancy: incidence and effect on outcome. Am J Obstet Gynecol 2002;186:77–83.

[7] Dickey RP, Gasser RF. Ultrasound evidence for variability in the size and development of normal human embryos before the tenth post-insemination week following assisted reproductive technologies. Hum Reprod 1993;8:331–7.

[8] Dickey RP, Sartor BM, Pyrzak R. No single outcome measure is satisfactory when evaluating success in assisted reproduction: both twin births and singleton births should be counted as successes. Hum Reprod 2004;19:783–7.

[9] Brenner WE, Edelman DA, Brazie JT. A standard of fetal growth for the United States of American. Am J Obstet Gynecol 1976;126:555–64.

[10] Evans MI, Dommergues M, Wapner RJ, et al. Efficacy of transabdominal multifetal pregnancy reduction: collaborative experience among the world's largest centers. Obstet Gynecol 1993;82: 61–6.

[11] Evans MI, Berkowitz RL, Wapner RJ, et al. Improvement in outcomes of multifetal pregnancy reduction with increased experience. Am J Obstet Gynecol 2001;184:97–103.

[12] Boulot P, Vignal J, Vergnes C, et al. Multifetal reduction of triplets to twins: a prospective comparison of pregnancy outcome. Hum Reprod 2000;15:1619–23.

[13] Alexander JM, Hammond KR, Steinkamph MP. Multifetal reduction of high-order multiple pregnancy: comparison of obstetrical outcome with nonreduced twin gestations. Fertil Steril 1995;64:1201–3.

[14] Groutz A, Yovel I, Amit A, et al. Pregnancy outcome after multifetal pregnancy reduction to twins compared with spontaneously conceived twins. Hum Reprod 1996;11:1334–6.

[15] Depp R, Macones GA, Rosenn MF, et al. Multifetal pregnancy reduction: evaluation of fetal growth in the remaining twins. Am J Obstet Gynecol 1996;174:1233–8.

[16] Torok O, Lapinski R, Salafia CM, et al. Multifetal pregnancy reduction is not associated with an increased risk of intrauterine growth restriction, except for very-high-order multiples. Am J Obstet Gynecol 1998;179:221–5.

[17] Smith-Levitin M, Kowalik A, Birnholz J, et al. Selective reduction of multifetal pregnancies to twins improves outcome over nonreduced triplet gestations. Am J Obstet Gynecol 1996;175:878–82.

[18] Macones GA, Schemmer G, Pritts E, et al. Multifetal reduction of triplets to twins improves perinatal outcome. Am J Obstet Gynecol 1993;169:982–6.

[19] Melgar C, Rosenfeld DL, Rawlinson K, et al. Perinatal outcome after multifetal reduction to twins compared with nonreduced multiple gestations. Obstet Gynecol 1991;78:763–7.

ELSEVIER
SAUNDERS

Obstet Gynecol Clin N Am
32 (2005) 29–38

OBSTETRICS AND
GYNECOLOGY
CLINICS
OF NORTH AMERICA

Neonatal Morbidity of Very Low Birth Weight Infants from Multiple Pregnancies

Eric S. Shinwell, MD

Department of Neonatology, Kaplan Medical Center, PO Box 1, Rehovot 76100, Jerusalem, Israel

Advances in perinatal and neonatal care in recent years have resulted in dramatic improvements in the rate of intact survival of preterm infants. As a result, neonatologists have focused on the new challenge of bringing about similar advances for the tiniest infants who are born at or near the current limits of viability. Although these tiny infants comprise only a small proportion of all births, the ravages of prematurity make them by far the most challenging group of infants who require our attention in the neonatal intensive care unit. Accordingly, when assigned to review the neonatal outcome of infants from multiple pregnancies in comparison to singletons, it seems appropriate to focus on those who are at highest risk for significant morbidity and mortality, namely very low birth weight (VLBW) and extremely low birth weight infants.

In view of the limitations of gestational age assessment, these infants are usually classified according to birth weight, in which VLBW refers to infants with a birth weight less than 1500 g. An important subset is termed "extremely low birth weight," which comprises infants with birth weight less than 1000 g, who are at particularly high risk.

VLBW infants may suffer from manifestations that result from their premature birth in all body systems, most commonly cardiorespiratory, neurologic, and gastrointestinal. Respiratory problems affect most of the infants and include respiratory distress syndrome and apnea of prematurity in the short term and bronchopulmonary dysplasia (BPD) or chronic lung disease in the long term. Despite the major advances in recent years related to widespread antenatal corticosteroids and postnatal surfactant, BPD still may persist in up to 20% of VLBW and 40% of extremely low birth weight infants at term age [1]. In the

E-mail address: eric_s@clalit.org.il

0889-8545/05/$ – see front matter © 2005 Elsevier Inc. All rights reserved.
doi:10.1016/j.ogc.2004.10.004
obgyn.theclinics.com

most severe cases, chronic respiratory insufficiency may continue into childhood, with a need for oxygen, medications, and frequent hospital admissions that may be related to exacerbations of the condition or secondary infection. Neurologic problems characteristic of VLBW infants include intraventricular hemorrhage (IVH) and periventricular leukomalacia. In recent years, the incidence and severity of IVH has decreased in most units, although it is still seen in approximately 15% to 20% of these infants [2]. Periventricular leukomalacia is seen less often (4%–8% in most series), with peak incidence at approximately 28 to 29 weeks' gestation, in contrast with the incidence of IVH, which seems to correlate inversely with gestational age [3]. Both of these conditions predispose to long-term neurodevelopmental impairment that may include cerebral palsy, mental retardation, and visual, hearing, and behavioral problems [4]. Recently, researchers have recognized that these sequelae may develop despite a normal head ultrasound examination and that MRI may advance our understanding of the relationship between neonatal central nervous system abnormality and neuro-developmental outcome [3]. Sepsis—vertically transmitted and nosocomial—is of particular concern in the immunocompromised extremely low birth weight infant; it affects 20% to 50% of these infants, 10% to 20% of whom may succumb [2]. Other major morbidities commonly seen in these infants include feeding difficulties, necrotizing enterocolitis, patent ductus arteriosus, and retino-pathy of prematurity. The mortality rate to discharge for VLBW infants in the United States is approximately 13% to 15% in recent series, although there is much variation among centers [5].

The epidemic of very low birth weight infants from multiple pregnancies

The evolution of assisted reproductive techniques and ovulation-induction therapy has resulted in an epidemic of multiple pregnancies over the last two decades. This growth has been coupled with the trend toward advanced maternal age in Western society [6,7]. In the United States between 1980 and 2001, twin births rose by 59% and higher-order multiple births rose by more than 400% [6]. Similarly, dramatic findings have been reported from Britain, Denmark, Canada, and Israel [8–11]. In recent years, although the twin birth rate has continued to rise each year, there seemed to be the beginnings of a leveling-off of the triplet birth rate during 1999 to 2001 [12]. It is unclear whether this represents a reduction in the number of high multiple pregnancies or increased use of multi-fetal pregnancy reduction; however, these changes clearly signify awareness among health care providers that multiple pregnancy should be regarded as a serious complication of ART [13].

The mean gestational age at birth is inversely correlated to plurality. In a large study of births in the United States, mean gestational age was 39 weeks in singletons, 35.8 weeks in twins, and 32.5 weeks in triplets [14]. The relationship between preterm delivery and birth weight in multiples also is complex because intrauterine growth in multiples is similar to that seen in singletons until approximately 22 weeks' gestation, when a small divergence becomes much more marked at approximately 28 weeks. Infants from multiple pregnancies are often more premature and smaller for gestational age than singletons.

The epidemic of infants from multiple births translates into an epidemic of VLBW infants. The combination of this increase in numbers, together with increasingly complex care that results in increased survival of tiny infants, has brought about a disproportionate increase in the workload of neonatal intensive care units. For example, infants from multiple pregnancies currently comprise 3% of all births in the United States [15]. Approximately half of the infants in the Israel VLBW neonatal database are the product of multiple pregnancies [11]. If this increased workload is not matched by appropriate staffing, quality of care may be affected [16].

Delivery room care

Researchers have suggested that the risks for VLBW infants from multiple births, particularly higher-order multiples, may be affected by altered behavior of the caregivers during the stressful minutes around the delivery. This behavior may be to the benefit or detriment of the infants. For example, if there is inadequate staff or equipment to cope with several high-risk infants, the result

Table 1
Recommended minimum staffing and equipment requirements for multiple births

Staff & equipment	Requirements
Delivery / operating room	
Pediatricians	One per infant (preferably more), all trained in neonatal resuscitation (preferably neonatal resuscitation program certified)
Supervising / back-up physician	At least one qualified neonatologist
Obstetricians	Must be alert to importance of the pediatric team being fully prepared before beginning delivery/operation
Nurses / midwives	One per infant, all trained in neonatal resuscitation
Radiant warmer	One per infant, preferably with servo temperature control
Resuscitation equipment per infant	Oxygen, ventilation bag, suction, laryngoscope, endotracheal tubes (various sizes), medications and other equipment; adequate space (often limited in operating rooms)
Temperature control	Operating room temperature at 24–26°C to minimize ambient heat loss, which may be a little uncomfortable for the staff
Transport incubators	One per infant
NICU	
Staff	As previously stated, plus back-up available for procedures
Radiant warmer / incubators	One per infant (not those from the delivery room)
Equipment	Prepared in advance of delivery for each infant; ventilators, monitors, sterile equipment for procedures (eg, umbilical lines), intravenous fluids

may be suboptimal care. The reverse also may be true, however, via different mechanisms. The excitement associated with higher-order births, in particular, often attracts many additional staff members. In order not to risk stressful situations in the noisy, crowded delivery or operating room, neonatologists also may opt to electively intubate extremely preterm infants and administer prophylactic surfactant therapy. This prophylactic approach, although controversial in older preterm infants, has been shown to decrease pneumothorax and neonatal mortality in extremely preterm infants [17].

As a recommendation for the care of higher-order multiples around the time of delivery, Table 1 offers suggested minimum requirements in terms of staffing and equipment for this situation.

Very low birth weight multiples: risks compared with singletons

Twins and higher-order multiples are at increased risk for perinatal and neonatal mortality (Table 2). This risk has been shown consistently in large population-based studies and single center reports with differing levels of care [18,19]. For example, recent data on all US births showed the neonatal mortality rate per 1000 live births to be 6.6 for singletons, 32 for twins, and as high as 71.8 for triplets [18]. Although absolute numbers vary among reports, the relative risks are mostly consistent. Luke and Keith [19] found the relative risk for VLBW to be 9.6 and 32.7 and for infant mortality to be 6.6 and 19.4, respectively, when comparing twins and triplets with singletons. A study from the Japanese vital statistics database showed the relative risk for perinatal mortality to be 5-fold and 12-fold higher for twins and triplets, respectively, compared with singletons [20].

Certain authors have claimed that aggressive modern perinatal and neonatal care may close the gap between the mortality risks of singletons, twins, and triplets, however. Single-center studies by Collins et al [21], Gonen et al [22], Sassoon et al [23], Angel et al [24], Ron-El et al [25], and Boulot et al [26] have reported excellent outcomes for infants from twin and higher-order multiple pregnancies. These studies have contributed to recognition of the possible benefits of aggressive antenatal and perinatal care in high-risk pregnancies. This research approach does not offer useful information in assessing the biologic

Table 2
Summary outcomes (compared to very low birth weight singletons)

Type of comparison	Outcome	Twins	Triplets
Unadjusted	RDS, BPD, IVH	↑	↑↑
	Mortality	↑	↑↑
	Cerebral palsy	↑	↑↑
Corrected for gestational age	Morbidity + mortality	Conflicting reports	
Corrected for case mix	Morbidity	=	=
	Mortality	=	↑

Abbreviation: RDS, respiratory distress syndrome.

risks of twins and higher-order multiples, however, but rather reflects issues in health care provision.

Comparisons of outcome after adjustment for gestational age

In view of the large differences in gestational age at birth between singletons, twins, and higher-order multiples, several authors have conducted comparative studies that have corrected for this important variable. Ballabh et al [27], Suri et al [28], Nielsen et al [29], and Maayan-Metzger et al [30] have reported on single-center analyses of samples varying in size from 128 to 1481 infants, with the number of sets of triplets in each study varying between 18 and 116. In these studies, although twins and triplets had small differences in the occurrence of certain variables, such as delivery by cesarean section and the incidence of retinopathy of prematurity, no significant differences were found in the incidence of major morbidity and mortality.

By comparison, Synnes et al [31] reported a single center study that focused on gestational age–corrected analyses of outcome in infants born at 23 to 28 weeks' gestation and found that twins had higher mortality rate at each week of gestation. Buekens and Wilcox [32] used a unique approach to adjusted comparisons by using z-scores for birth weight–corrected analyses, thereby accounting for the variation in growth patterns between singletons and twins. In this large, population-based study ($n = 234,292$), twins were found to have higher mortality rates over the whole range of birth weights. Ericson et al [33] found similar results in Swedish infants from 1973 to 1988. More recently, Jacquemyn et al [34] compared morbidity and mortality in singletons and twins from Flanders from 1998 to 1999. Twins of 24 to 27 weeks' gestation had higher neonatal mortality rates than singletons. In other gestational age groups, however, no differences were found in morbidity or mortality.

The conclusions of these studies are limited, however, by the marked differences between the study groups in potential confounding variables, such as use of fertility treatments, maternal age and ethnicity, intrauterine growth retardation, antenatal corticosteroid administration, and mode of delivery.

Comparisons of outcome after adjustment for confounding variables

Single center studies, such as those of Kaufman et al [35], reported relatively small samples. After correction for confounders, however, no significant differences were found between singletons, twins, and triplets in mortality and major morbidity. Stewart et al [36] focused on abnormalities on cranial ultrasound in VLBW singletons, twins, and triplets. After correction for relevant confounders, no significant differences were found between the groups, but a slightly lower incidence of IVH was noted in infants conceived by assisted reproductive techniques as compared with infants conceived spontaneously.

To improve the comparability of the study groups in research on the effects of plurality, it is important to adjust appropriately for as many potential confounding variables as possible and to make use of large samples. One such study was reported by Donovan et al [37] in the neonatal research network of the National Institute of Child Health and Development. This study compared the outcomes of singletons and twins (without higher-order multiples) in a sample of 10,271 VLBW infants from 12 tertiary neonatal referral centers. Twins comprised almost 20% of all VLBW infants admitted during the study period, and mothers of twins received more prenatal care and more antenatal steroids than mothers of singletons. Twin infants were more often delivered by cesarean section, suffered more often from respiratory distress syndrome, and required more surfactant. After correction for these confounding variables, however, no statistically significant differences were found between singletons and twins in mortality or in the incidence of major morbidity such as BPD or IVH.

Another large study that focused on VLBW multiples and added triplets to the previous comparison was conducted by the Israeli VLBW neonatal database. This continuing project collects and studies extensive perinatal and neonatal information on VLBW infants born in all of the country's 28 neonatal intensive care units [38]. In this study, major adverse outcomes were compared between singletons and complete sets of twins and triplets that were VLBW and were born alive at 24 to 32 weeks' gestation. As with the study by the National Institute of Child Health and Development, marked differences were found between the groups in the incidence of important confounding perinatal variables, and multiple logistic regression analyses were performed to assess the independent contribution of plurality. The sample included 3717 singletons (66%), 1394 twins (25%), and 483 triplets (9%) born between 1995 and 1999. Use of assisted reproductive techniques was found in 10% of singletons, 56% of twins, and 91% of triplets. Mothers of twins and triplets were significantly more likely to begin antenatal care in the first trimester and receive antenatal steroids. Delivery by caesarean section was more common in triplets (89%) than in twins (65%) or singletons (62%). A small inverse correlation was found between gestational age and birth weight (singletons: gestational age 28.9 ± 2.6 weeks, birth weight 1096 ± 269 g; twins: gestational age 28.4 ± 2.3 weeks, birth weight 1062 ± 271 g; triplets: gestational age 28.5 ± 2.4 weeks, birth weight 1049 ± 259 g). Another important difference between the study groups involved the incidence of infants who were small for gestational age. Among singletons, 28.8% were small for gestational age compared with 15.5% and 16.4% of twins and triplets, respectively. This finding probably reflects the different causes for preterm labor in these groups. Twins and triplets are born early primarily because of lack of space, whereas in singletons premature labor often reflects growth and development problems in utero.

Respiratory distress syndrome was significantly more common in twins (70%; OR 1.58, 95% CI 1.32–1.89) and triplets (75%; OR 2.51, 95% CI 1.87–3.37) compared with singletons (60%), and it occurred despite higher exposure to antenatal steroids in these two groups. Researchers previously suggested that the effect of antenatal steroids in multiples may be less than in singletons or even may be absent. This effect is also influenced by race, with the maximal effect seen in singleton, black infants; thus, the predominantly white origin of the Israeli sample may contribute to this finding [39].

On univariate analysis, no significant differences were found between the groups regarding the incidence of the major adverse outcomes—chronic lung disease, adverse neurologic findings (severe IVH, periventricular leukomalacia, or ventricular dilatation), or death. Multivariate logistic regression analysis, which accounts for the relevant confounding variables, found triplets to be at significantly increased risk for mortality compared with twins and singletons (OR 1.54, 95% CI 1.13–2.11). The risk for chronic lung disease and adverse neurologic findings was similar in all groups.

Both of these large studies have concluded that even after careful adjustment for differences in case mix there seem to be no significant differences between singletons and twins in neonatal morbidity and mortality. By comparison, there may be an increased risk for mortality in triplets that awaits confirmation from other large, carefully conducted studies.

Effect of birth order

It has long been thought that second-born twins are at increased risk for neonatal respiratory and other morbidity and perhaps even mortality [40]. Certain studies have postulated that these risks may result from a degree of perinatal asphyxia secondary to malpresentation and delay in delivery of the second twin, in particular in vaginal deliveries [41]. Perinatal and neonatal care practices that may influence these findings have changed profoundly in recent years. The widespread use of antenatal glucocorticoids and postnatal surfactant therapy has reduced dramatically the incidence and severity of respiratory distress syndrome, IVH, and mortality in VLBW infants. The incidence of delivery by cesarean section also continues to rise and is approximately 70% for all VLBW infants and even higher for multiples [2]. In view of these developments, the issue of the risks of the VLBW second twin has been revisited in recent studies.

A large recent study was based on the Israel National VLBW infant database with methodology as described previously [42]. The study included a population-based sample of 1328 twins born during 1995 to 1999. Approximately 80% of twin pairs were concordant for neonatal morbidity and mortality. Second twins were found to be at increased risk for respiratory distress syndrome, however (OR 1.51, 95% CI 1.29–1.76), BPD (OR 1.36, 95% CI 1.11–1.66), and death (OR 1.24, 95% CI 1.02–1.51) but not for adverse neurologic findings (OR 1.20, 95% CI 0.91–1.60) when compared with first-born twins. Although second twins had increased risk for malpresentation, the mode of delivery did not significantly influence outcome. The increased risk for respiratory distress syndrome and BPD was found in vaginal and cesarean deliveries.

The influence of birth order on BPD may be short-lived, because studies by Hacking et al [43] and Donovan et al [37] reported no difference between the twins in BPD at 36 weeks' gestation corrected gestational age as compared with age 28 days as reported earlier.

In a recent large population-based study, Sheay et al [44] found increased breech presentation, fetal distress, cesarean delivery, and perinatal mortality in second-born twins. The increased mortality was primarily related to increased stillbirths, however, and no difference was found in neonatal or post-neonatal mortality between first- and second-born twins at any stage of gestation. This study did not report on neonatal morbidity.

Summary

In the era of antenatal steroids and postnatal surfactant, although VLBW twins are concordant for most outcomes, second-born twins remain at increased risk for respiratory morbidity. Regarding other morbidities and mortality, further studies are required to clarify the issue.

References

[1] Martin RJ, Walsh-Sukys MC. Bronchopulmonary dysplasia: no simple solution. N Engl J Med 1999;340:1036–8.

[2] Fanaroff AA, Hack M, Walsh MC. The NICHD neonatal research network: changes in practice and outcomes during the first 15 years. Semin Perinatol 2003;27(4):281–7.

[3] Inder TE, Anderson NJ, Spencer C, et al. White matter injury in the premature infant: a comparison between serial cranial sonographic and MR findings at term. AJNR Am J Neuroradiol 2003;24(5):805–9.

[4] Hack M, Flannery DJ, Schluchter M, et al. Outcomes in young adulthood for very low birth weight infants. N Engl J Med 2002;346:149–57.

[5] Lemons JA, Bauer CR, Oh W, et al. Very low birth weight outcomes of the National Institute of Child Health and Human Development neonatal research network, January 1995 through December 1996. NICHD Neonatal Research Network. Pediatrics 2001;107(1):E1–8.

[6] MacDorman MF, Minino AM, Strobino DM, et al. Annual summary of vital statistics: 2001. Pediatrics 2002;110:1037–52.

[7] Division of Reproductive Health, National Center for Chronic Disease Prevention and Health Promotion. Contribution of assisted reproductive technology and ovulation-inducing drugs to triplet and higher-order multiple births: United States, 1980–1997. MMWR Morb Mortal Wkly Rep 2000;49:535–8.

[8] Doyle P. The outcome of multiple pregnancy. Hum Reprod 1996;11:110–7.

[9] Westergaard T, Wohlfahrt J, Aaby P, et al. Population based study of rates of multiple pregnancies in Denmark, 1980–94. BMJ 1997;314:775–9.

[10] Millar WJ, Wadhera S, Nimrod C. Multiple births: trends and patterns in Canada, 1974–90. Health Rep 1992;4(3):223–50.

[11] Reichman B. Israel national very low birth weight infant database. Jerusalem: Israel Ministry of Health Publication; 2003.

[12] Martin JA, Hamilton BE, Ventura SJ, et al. Births: final data for 2001. National Vital Statistics Reports 2002;51(2):1–102.

[13] Adashi EY, Ekins MN, La Coursiere Y. On the discharge of Hippocratic' obligations: challenges and opprtunities. Am J Ob Gyn 2004;190:885–93.

[14] Alexander GR, Kogen M, Martin J, et al. What are the fetal growth patterns of singletons, twins and triplets in the United States? Clin Obstet Gynecol 1998;41(1):115–25.

[15] Guyer B, Hoyert DL, Martin JA, et al. Annual summary of vital statistics: 1998. Pediatrics 1999;104:1229–46.

[16] Tucker J, Tarnow-Mordi W, Gould C, et al. UK neonatal intensive care services in 1996: on behalf of the UK Neonatal Staffing Study Collaborative Group. Arch Dis Child Fetal Neonatal Ed 1999;80(3):F233–4.

[17] Horbar JD, Carpenter JH, Buzas J, et al. Vermont Oxford Network Timing of initial surfactant treatment for infants 23 to 29 weeks' gestation: is routine practice evidence based? Pediatrics 2004;113(6):1593–602.

[18] Martin JA, Park MM. Trends in twin and triplet births: 1980–1997. Natl Vital Stat Rep 1999; 47(24):1–16.

[19] Luke B, Keith L. The contribution of singletons, twins and triplets to low birth weight, infant mortality and handicap in the United States. J Reprod Med 1992;37:661–5.

[20] Imaizumi Y. Perinatal morality in triplet births in Japan: trends and factors influencing mortality. Twin Res 2003;6:1–6.

[21] Collins JW, Merrick D, David RJ, et al. The Northwestern University Triplet Study III: Neonatal outcome. Acta Genet Med Gemellol 1988;37(1):77–80.

[22] Gonen R, Heyman E, Asztalos EV, et al. The outcome of triplet, quadruplet and quintuplet pregnancies managed in a perinatal unit: obstetric, neonatal and follow-up data. Am J Obstet Gynecol 1990;162(2):454–9.

[23] Sassoon DA, Castro LC, Davis JL, et al. Perinatal outcome in triplet versus twin gestations. Obstet Gynecol 1990;75(5):817–20.

[24] Angel JL, Kalter CS, Morales WJ, et al. Aggressive perinatal care for high-order multiple gestations: does good perinatal outcome justify aggressive assisted reproductive techniques? Am J Obstet Gynecol 1999;181(2):253–9.

[25] Ron-El R, Mor Z, Weinraub Z, et al. Triplet, quadruplet and quintuplet pregnancies: management and outcome. Acta Obstet Gynecol Scand 1992;71(5):347–50.

[26] Boulot P, Hedon B, Pelliccia G, et al. Favourable outcome in 33 triplet pregnancies managed between 1985–90. Eur J Obstet Gynecol Reprod Biol 1992;43(2):123–9.

[27] Ballabh P, Kumari J, Al Kouatly HB, et al. Neonatal outcome of triplet versus twin and singleton pregnancies: a matched case control study. Eur J Obstet Gynecol Reprod Biol 2003;107:28–36.

[28] Suri K, Bhandari V, Lerer T, et al. Morbidity and mortality of preterm twins and higher-order multiple births. J Perinatol 2001;21:293–9.

[29] Nielsen H, Harvey-Wilkes K, MacKinnon B, et al. Neonatal outcome of very premature infants from multiple and singleton gestations. Am J Obstet Gynecol 1997;177:653–9.

[30] Maayan Metzger A, Naor N, Sirota L. Comparative outcome study between triplet and singleton infants. Acta Pediatr 2002;91:1208–11.

[31] Synnes AR, Ling EWY, Whitfield MF, et al. Perinatal outcomes of a large cohort of extremely low gestational age infants (twenty-three to twenty-eight completed weeks of gestation). J Pediatr 1994;125:952–60.

[32] Buekens P, Wilcox A. Why do small twins have a lower mortality rate than small singletons? Am J Obstet Gynecol 1993;168:937–41.

[33] Ericson A, Gunnarskog J, Kallen B, et al. A registry study of very low birthweight liveborn infants in Sweden, 1973–1988. Acta Obstet Gynecol Scand 1992;71(2):104–11.

[34] Jacquemyn Y, Martens G, Ruyssinck G, et al. A matched cohort comparison of the outcome of twin versus singleton pregnancies in Flanders, Belgium. Twin Res 2003;6:7–11.

[35] Kaufman GE, Malone FD, Harvey-Wilkes KB, et al. Neonatal morbidity and mortality associated with triplet pregnancy. Obstet Gynecol 1998;91(3):342–8.

[36] Stewart JE, Allred EN, Collins M, et al. Risk of cranial ultrasound abnormalities in very low birth weight infants conceived with assisted reproductive techniques. J Perinatol 2002;22:37–45.

[37] Donovan EF, Ehrenkrantz RA, Shankaran S, et al. Outcomes of very low birth weight twins cared for in the National Institute of Child Health and Human Development Neonatal Research Network's intensive care units. Am J Obstet Gynecol 1998;179:742–9.

[38] Shinwell ES, Blickstein I, Lusky A, et al, in collaboration with the Israel Neonatal Network. Excess risk of mortality in very low birthweight triplets: a national, population-based study. Arch Dis Child Fetal Neonatal Ed 2003;88:F36–40.

[39] Quist Therson EC, Myhr TL, Ohlsson A. Antenatal steroids to prevent respiratory distress syndrome: multiple gestation as an effect modifier. Acta Obstet Gynecol Scand 1999;78(5):388–92.

[40] Ellis RF, Berger GS, Keith L, et al. The Northwestern University Multihospital Twin Study. II. Mortality of first versus second twins. Acta Genet Med Gemellol 1979;28(4):347–52.

[41] Arnold C, McLean FH, Kramer MS, et al. Respiratory distress syndrome in second-born versus first-born twins: a matched case-control analysis. N Engl J Med 1987;317:1121–5.

[42] Shinwell ES, Blickstein I, Lusky A, et al, in collaboration with the Israel Neonatal Network. The effect of birth order on neonatal morbidity and mortality among very low birth weight twins: a population-based study. Arch Dis Child Fetal Neonatal Ed 2004;89(2):F145–8.

[43] Hacking D, Watkins A, Fraser S, et al, on behalf of Australia and New Zealand Neonatal Network. Respiratory distress syndrome and birth order in premature twins. Arch Dis Child Fetal Neonatal Ed 2001;84:F117–21.

[44] Sheay W, Ananth CV, Kinzler WJ. Perinatal mortality in first and second born twins in the United States. Obstet Gynecol 2004;103:63–7.

ELSEVIER
SAUNDERS

Obstet Gynecol Clin N Am
32 (2005) 39–54

OBSTETRICS AND
GYNECOLOGY
CLINICS
OF NORTH AMERICA

Growth Aberration in Multiple Pregnancy

Isaac Blickstein, MD[a,b,*]

[a]*Department of Obstetrics and Gynecology, Kaplan Medical Center, 76100 Rehovot, Israel*
[b]*Hadassah-Hebrew University School of Medicine, Jerusalem, Israel*

Most recent US data show that 10.2% of twins and 34.5% of triplets weigh less than 1500 g at birth (very low birth weight [VLBW] infants) [1]. These figures are practically the same as those reported by Alexander et al [2] for the period 1991 to 1995, and they represent more than 9-fold and more than 30-fold higher percentages of VLBW twin and triplet infants compared with singletons. No special mathematical skills are required to calculate that twin and triplet infants comprise more than 25% of the population of VLBW infants born in the United States in 2002 [1]. The significance of this number is even more striking given that US twins and triplets comprise approximately 3.3% of all neonates.

Because the human female is "programmed" by nature to carry one fetus at a time (as is the case in 99% of spontaneous human conceptions), the fact that multiples weigh less than singleton neonates is not surprising, nor is it surprising that the mean birth weight decreases with increasing plurality. Fig. 1 shows the relationship between mean birth weight and plurality, which satisfies a perfect ($R^2 = 0.999$) polynomial function ($Y = 132X^2 - 1342X + 4529$, where Y is birth weight and X is number of infants).

The comparison between multiples and singletons in terms of intrauterine growth is more complex than it seems at first glance. Essentially, it is not true that multiples grow differently throughout gestation. In fact, birth weights by gestational age curves, the so-called "growth curves", clearly demonstrate that singletons, twins, and triplets grow similarly until 28 weeks' gestation, when the curve of multiples begins to deviate from that of singletons. With more advanced gestational ages, a second point of deviation may be observed, at approximately 35 weeks' gestation, when the curve of triplets begins to deviate from that of

* Department of Obstetrics and Gynecology, Kaplan Medical Center, 76100 Rehovot, Israel.
E-mail address: blick@netvision.net.il

0889-8545/05/$ – see front matter © 2005 Elsevier Inc. All rights reserved.
doi:10.1016/j.ogc.2004.10.006

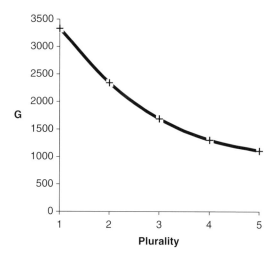

Fig. 1. Relationship between mean birth weight and plurality. (*Data from* Martin JA, Hamilton BE, Sutton PD, et al. Births: final data for 2002. Natl Vital Stat Rep 2003;52:1–113.)

twins (Fig. 2). These dates coincide with changes in other important milestones in the in utero development of multiples.

Function of the utero-placental unit

Fetal growth is determined by constitutional characteristics modulated by the function of the utero-placental unit. The constitutional determinants explain the variance of normal human fetuses and why not all small-for-gestational-age (SGA) infants result from an intrauterine growth restriction process. The function

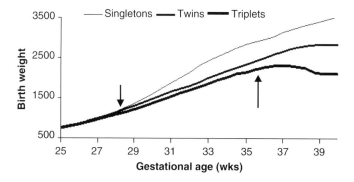

Fig. 2. Growth curves of singletons, twins, and triplets show the deviation of multiples' curves from the singleton's curve at 28 weeks' gestation (*left arrow*) and the deviation of the triplets' curve from the twins' curve at 35 to 36 weeks' gestation (*right arrow*). (*Adapted from* Alexander GR, Kogan M, Martin J, et al. What are the fetal growth patterns of singletons, twins, and triplets in the United States? Clin Obstet Gynecol 1998;41:114–25; with permission.)

of the utero-placental unit, on the other hand, determines the extent of the expression of the underlying genetic factors by controlling transfer of oxygen and nutrients. Damage to the utero-placental unit predictably restricts fetal growth (as is the case with several types of infection and maternal disease conditions), although the fetus may or may not be SGA.

An appropriately functioning utero-placental unit is expected to provide for an increase in fetal mass according to the underlying fetal constitutional characteristics. Normal singletons grow in utero at a predictable growth rate, and the uterine size adjusts to contain the growing gestation. Put differently, uterine size is infrequently a restricting factor for fetal growth; on the contrary, the uterus normally adjusts to a larger-than-expected content by the well-known phenomenon of overdistension. Such an adjustment to the mismatch between the size of gestation and the size of the uterus is not unlimited. When the uterus exceeds its limited capacity to distend, contractions often ensue, and when these contractions occur prematurely, they may lead to preterm labor and delivery. In such a construct, the larger the plurality, and the greater uterine content, the lower the gestational age. No wonder that the pattern shown in Fig. 1 for birth weight duplicates the relationship between the mean gestational age at birth and plurality shown in Fig. 3, which also satisfies perfect ($R^2 = 0.999$) polynomial functions ($Y = 0.36X^2 - 47X + 43.2$, where Y equals gestational age and X equals number of infants).

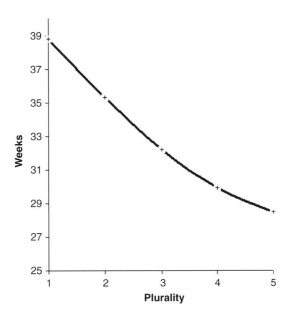

Fig. 3. Relationship between mean gestational age and plurality. (*Data from* Martin JA, Hamilton BE, Sutton PD, et al. Births: final data for 2002. Natl Vital Stat Rep 2003;52:1–113.)

Ideally, it follows that the utero-placental unit provides for fetal size (birth weight) and fetal maturity (gestational age). Whereas size and maturity of singletons increase in parallel, this is practically impossible in multiple pregnancies, because the total size of the gestations gradually exceeds the normal uterine size of a singleton.

Uterine adaptation to supplying sufficient nutrition for the excess fetal mass in multiple gestations is invariably required as early as the beginning of the second half of the pregnancy. The incredible metabolic changes in a multiple pregnancy are appreciated when one considers that the median birth weight of a singleton (3289 g) is achieved by a pair of twins as early as 31 weeks' gestation, when the median of the total fetal birth weight (both twins) is 3358 g. In triplets, the median singleton birth weight at 40 weeks' gestation is attained by the three fetuses combined even earlier, at 28 weeks [3]. Put differently, if the utero-placental unit should be required to provide the median singleton birth weight at 38 weeks' gestation for the entire twin or triplet pregnancy, then the resulting average birth weight of a twin or a triplet would be only 1650 g and 1100 g, respectively. The individual birth weights of twins and triplets at that gestational age far exceed these values.

Several more recent observations support these findings. For example, a comparison between the total birth weight of a multiple pregnancy to the ninetieth percentile—the so-called "large-for-gestational-age" or "macrosomic" singleton—during the third trimester shows that between 28 and 38 weeks' gestation, the entire fetal mass of twin pairs and triplet sets exceeds that of a macrosomic singleton [3]. The total triplet birth weight of more than 99% of triplet sets delivered at more than 32 weeks' gestation is heavier than any large-for-gestational-age singleton delivered at more than 35 weeks, which implies that triplets delivered by 32 weeks' gestation were nurtured by a uterine milieu that is definitely performing in its full capacity [3]. At 30 to 32 weeks' gestation, the uterine milieu is probably performing in its full capacity because at least 80% of the triplet sets delivered at this stage had a total weight more than the macrosomic singleton at 40 weeks. Conversely, it seems that the uterine environment is less efficient before 30 weeks' gestation. It is possible that some triplets are delivered before 30 weeks because the uterine milieu is not performing in its full capacity [3]. Finally, the utero-placental unit is still efficient even in cases of severely discordant twins [4]. When the "excess fetal mass" in more than 25% of discordant twins ($n = 12,846$) is compared with the median birth weight of singletons at less than 28 weeks' gestation, the utero-placental unit produces more than 75% of "fetal mass" compared with singletons. With advanced gestation, the excess mass gradually decreases to approximately 50%, a value that remains relatively unchanged until approximately 37 weeks, when it declines again [4]. This observation suggests that even when severe discordance is present in twin pregnancies, the utero-placental unit supplies 50% to 75% more than for the average singleton gestation.

The human uterine milieu limits the growth potential of the individual fetus in a multiple pregnancy, and as a rule, third-trimester multiples are likely to be growth restricted compared with singletons. At the same time, however, the entire multiple pregnancy is growth promoted rather than restricted [3].

Intrauterine growth restriction and small-for-gestational-age status in multiples

Growth-restricted infants, by definition, are infants who fail to grow according to their growth potential. Because all third-trimester multiples are likely to be growth restricted compared with singletons, it follows that the growth potential of multiples and singletons are not the same. Within the uterine constrains, twins and triplets have different growth rates than singletons. Each member may grow at a different rate. For example, the individual mean triplet birth weights by gestational age regression lines show a highly significant linear correlation (Pearson's r-values, 0.996–0.998), but the comparisons of the regression slopes (ie, proxy for growth rate) among the largest, middle, and the smaller triplets were significantly different [5]. This observation suggests that each fetus in a triplet set may have its own linear growth pattern but with a significantly different inclination than that of its siblings [5].

Most students of fetal growth assess twins and triplets as singletons; therefore, many twins and almost all triplets are considered SGA by singleton standards. When the median birth weights of twins and triplets (who represent the average fetus) are compared with the tenth birth weight percentile of singletons (who represent the SGA or the so-called "potentially growth-restricted singleton"), however, the average twin is not SGA by singleton standards until approximately 38 weeks' gestation, and the average triplet is not SGA by singleton standards until approximately 35 weeks [3].

The ratio between the median birth weight of twin/singleton and triplet/singleton, which is elaborated by re-assessing the data presented by Alexander et al [2], produces a predictable pattern for the growth of a given member of a multiple pregnancy set compared with the (expected) growth of a singleton [3]. The patterns suggest four phases. In phase A, a ratio of 0.9 to 1.0 (ie, similar birth weights to singletons) is maintained until 28 and 30 weeks' gestation in triplets and twins, respectively. Phase B, which begins at 30 weeks in twins and earlier in triplets, demonstrates a steady decrease in birth weights of the individual multiple relative to singletons. During phase C, the ratio does not change significantly over time. Phase D, seen only in triplets, represents a marked decrease in triplet birth weight relative to singletons, when triplets make it to an advanced gestational age [3]. The data used in this analysis is cross-sectional rather than longitudinal. Two different uterine conditions are apparent. The first condition promotes age and maintains size (phases A and C), whereas the second condition promotes age and restricts size (phases B and D). Because all phases promote age, it seems that from an individual fetal perspective, nature favors advanced gestational age (ie, maturity) at the expense of size [3].

Another way to look at fetal growth is to evaluate the ponderal index (a measure of size rather than weight). When SGA triplets (less than the tenth percentile by triplets standards) were evaluated, approximately 70% did not have a low ponderal index, whereas 79.2% of infants with a low ponderal index were not SGA by triplet standards [6]. The study concluded that most triplets with a low ponderal index might not be considered growth restricted [6].

Sonography is accurate in following growth patterns of an individual fetus by using growth curves of either singleton or multiples. A distinction is made between a single sonographic observation and a longitudinal follow-up of fetal growth. In the former case, the fetus can be designated only as SGA and the estimated fetal weight should be compared with reference values found in various charts for twins and triplets [3]. Conversely, repeated bi-weekly sonography can establish whether growth is actually arrested and whether the SGA fetus is also growth restricted. Whenever an SGA fetus is observed in a multiple pregnancy, one should treat it as any SGA singleton.

Growth discordance

Birth weight discordance—the difference between the heaviest and the lightest fetus in a set of multiples—is common, because some variation is expected among siblings. Growth discordance has been associated with adverse outcomes, however, mainly because it is associated with growth restriction.

Numerous studies on discordance, especially in twin gestations, were published during the past 50 years. The specific cause is yet to be determined. The reason for discordance cannot be a rare condition, because otherwise it would be difficult to explain why this phenomenon is rather common. More plausible is the concept that birth weight discordance, at large, is a quasi-physiologic condition, the incidence of which decreases from approximately 30% at discordance level of less than 5% to less than 4% for discordance of 25% to 30% and further to less than 1% for discordance of more than 40% [4]. In other words, approximately 75% of twins exhibit less than 15% discordance, an additional 20% are 15% to 25% discordant, and approximately 5% are more than 25% discordant [4].

Some generalizations of the discordance phenomenon in twins have been suggested [4]. First, if discordance were a chance event, twin A and twin B would have the same chance of being the smaller one. Researchers have established that at levels of discordance less than 25%, either twin can be the smaller, but the likelihood of the second-born twin being the smaller increases with increasing discordance levels [7,8]. At a level more than 25%, the smaller twin is three to six times more often the second born [8]. Second, research recently suggested that in terms of neonatal mortality, the percent definition (>25%) and the ninety-fifth percentile of discordance by gestational age can be used interchangeably to define pairs at risk [4]. Third, not all discordant pairs are similar and some fare better than others. It seems that even among severely discordant twins there is a substantial group in which there is no genuine growth restriction [9]. In a recent study, 10,683 pairs that exhibited more than 25% discordance were classified according to the birth weight of the smaller twin, being less than tenth percentile (ie, SGA), tenth to fiftieth, or more than fiftieth percentile (ie, appropriate for gestational age). Only approximately 60% of these severely discordant twins were associated with an SGA twin. Consequently, the neonatal mortality rate was significantly higher among pairs in which the smaller twin weighed less than the tenth birth weight percentile, a difference that results from the higher mortality among the smaller but not among the larger twins [9]. Fourth, it seems that the likelihood for an adverse outcome is greater with larger discordance levels [10,11], which may result from the fact that discordant twins, especially at lower degrees of discordance, do not necessarily represent absolute growth restriction. Fifth, the same discordance level may have a different clinical implication in different gestational ages [11]. The cause of early size discordance might be different from third-trimester discordance. Finally, pairs affected by severe discordance (>25%) are at disproportionate risk for neonatal mortality when compared with concordant smaller or larger twins [12].

In triplets, higher frequency and severity of birth weight discordance is observed. Jones et al [13] found that 30.4% of 196 sets were more than 25% discordant, a figure similar to that found by others [14,15]. Large discordance levels (>40%) were found in 7% to 11.8% [13,15]. A much larger database found discordance levels of 25.1% to 35% and more than 35% in as many as 19.4% and 9.5% of the 2804 triplets analyzed, respectively, thrice higher than that found in twins [16]. These frequencies of discordance in triplets use the difference between the largest and smallest triplet of each set [13–15]. In this way, however, the middle-sized fetus is ignored, and as a result, the true intertriplet relationship is disregarded. A new description of discordance in triplets recently was proposed in which the relative birth weight of the middle triplet was defined [16]. Discordant sets were defined as (1) symmetrical when the birth weight of the middle fetus was within 25% of the average birth weight between the larger and smaller triplet, (2) low-skew when a set comprised one large and two small triplets, and (3) high-skew if the set comprised two large and one small triplet infants. The analysis showed that the three distinct types are gestational-age independent, with average frequencies of 57%, 30%, and 13%, for symmetrical, high-skew, and low-skew triplet sets, respectively. The data indicate that symmetrically discordant sets are probably the standard arrangement favored by the uterine environment and among discordant sets, one rather than two of the triplets was more often smaller [16]. Jacobs et al [17] independently proposed a similar approach and showed that increasing discordance level in triplets was associated with increased risk of fetal death and frequency of SGA infants.

The cutoff level of birth weight discordance, which differentiates between a normal variation and pathology, is still controversial. Most clinicians would agree, however, that a difference in birth weights of less than 25% is unlikely to be pathologic. Conversely, differences as high as 20% or 25% are also unlikely to represent a normal variation. In the last few years, several studies were conducted to describe a discordance model in relation to the uterine capacity to nurture twins. To avoid the potentially confounding effect of gestational age, the total twin birth weight was assumed to represent the capacity of the uterine environment to nurture twins at any given time. It follows that if discordance is a normal variation, similar frequencies of discordance are expected across total twin birth weights. The frequencies of birth weight discordance of more than 25% across the total twin birth weights decreased in a nonlinear, inversely logarithmic trend, however [8]. This observation suggests that the more favorable the uterine milieu (ie, larger total birth weight) for carrying twins, the smaller the likelihood of discordance. This conclusion was supported by showing that at a discordance level of 15% to 24.9%, the frequency function was inversely linear, as would have been expected with a normal variation [18]. At severe discordance levels of 25% to 34.9% and 35% or more, however, the patterns did not support a normal variation, because frequency functions were inversely logarithmic with a much steeper decrease at the level of 35% or more [18]. In clinical terms, these observations [8,18] support the concept that at levels of less than 25%, discordance seems to be related to a normal variation expected from the natural dissimilarities between siblings. Conversely, at levels more than 35%, discordance seems to be related to the exhausted uterine environment and reflects growth restriction.

For these two tails of the distribution (ie, those with lower and those with high levels of discordance), little controversy exists regarding the possible significance and the management options. Between these levels are twins (approximately 10% of the entire twin population) whose discordance cannot be explained by either a normal variation or growth restriction, however. This relative growth restriction within the framework of normal outcome can be explained by the concept of growth discordance as an adaptive measure to promote maturity. This hypothesis suggests that within a limited uterine environment, the combination of one larger and one smaller twin may reduce uterine overdistension and increase gestational age.

The indirect support of this assumption is that discordant twins (>25%) are delivered at a more advanced gestational age compared with concordant twins of the same total twin birth weight (representing the uterine volume) [19]. A comparison of pairs from the US Matched Multiple Birth Data File, grouped at intervals of 250 g total birth weight, found that the mean gestational age of discordant pairs was significantly higher across the entire range of total birth weights examined (<4750 g) [19].

Another indirect support to this hypothesis comes from the significant effect of parity on fetal growth in multiples, whereby significant differences exist between concordant and discordant pairs among primiparas, mainly at the lower birth weight strata [19]. The parity effect was similar in primiparas with triplets, who had significantly less concordant sets [16]. The notion that uterine volume affects growth of multiples is also supported by a large cohort of US live-born triplets, which shows a significant positive correlation ($R^2 = 0.95$) between the mean total triplet birth weight and maternal height [20]. Specifically, primiparas who were taller than 165 cm had age, body mass index, and gestational age characteristics similar to those of their shorter counterparts but delivered significantly heavier triplets and were at significantly lower risk of delivering VLBW triplets. In this case, maternal height represented the capacity of the uterus to expand during a multiple pregnancy.

In terms of frequency and severity, the apparent dissimilarity between discordance in twin and triplet gestations calls for a different conceptual approach to birth weight discordance in higher-order multiples. The polynomial function that describes the relationship between the frequencies of more than 25% discordant triplet sets and total birth weight deciles [16] is different from the inverse logarithmic relationship found in twins [8]. In clinical terms, the difference between the two functions is consistent with the difference between the uterine capacity in the two situations, but the general observation remains the same for twins and triplets: the more favorable the uterine milieu, the smaller the likelihood of discordant growth [16].

Management of growth aberrations in multiple pregnancies

Management of growth problems in twins and triplets is complex for two simple reasons. First, the diagnosis of a pathologic condition is often discordant. When such a condition is diagnosed remote from term, prompt delivery of the twin pair might be beneficial for the growth-restricted twin but exposes the normal co-twin to the risks of preterm birth. Second, and not the least important, is the potential error involved in the diagnosis of growth aberrations in multiples [21]. Fig. 4 shows the curves of a ±10% error in relation to the 0% error curve of sonographic estimates of birth weights. According to this curve and under the acceptable ±10% error, if both twins have the same birth weight (ie, absolutely concordant)—for example 2000 g—the estimated discordance might be as much 2200/1800 g (18.2%). If, on the other hand, the discordance level is 10% (2000/1800), the estimated difference within these sonographic margins of error might be 2200/1620 g or 26.4% discordance. True discordance also may be vastly underestimated. For example, suppose that 30% discordance exists (2000/1400 g). If the larger twin is underestimated and the smaller twin is overestimated by the ±10% error, the estimated discordance would be 1800/1540 g or 14.4% [21].

These pitfalls in assessing compared growth variables for predicting discordant growth in twin gestations lead to limited accuracy when held to a standard for discordance that requires intervention [21,22]. For example, Caravello et al [22] assessed the accuracy of estimating birth weight among twins with intrapair discordance of more than 25% and determined the relative accuracy of a difference in abdominal circumferences of 20 mm or more or estimated fetal weight of 25% or more. The authors found that the accuracy of predicting birth weight, as determined by mean error and percentage of the estimate within 10% of the actual weight, was similar between the discordant and nondiscordant pairs. Receiver-operating characteristic curves showed that diagnostic tests were under the nondiagnostic line. Most important, prediction limit calculations indicate that a

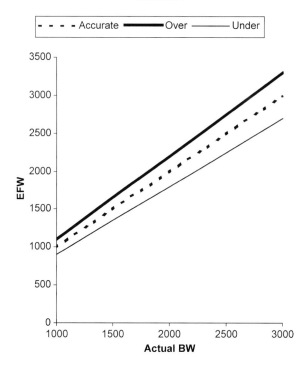

Fig. 4. Sonographic estimates of fetal weights compared with actual birth weight. The lines show the accurate estimation and over- and underestimations within a ±10% margin of error.

90% certainty that the actual birth weight discordance was at least 25% was achievable only if the difference in abdominal circumferences was 172 mm or more or the difference in estimated fetal weight was 112% or more.

Three additional points should be addressed. The first issue is related to early onset of discordance. If discordance is a result of some form of placental insufficiency, it is expected to begin during early third trimester. When discordance begins earlier, a meticulous search for other causes should be performed. One cause is discordant fetal anomaly, which may manifest as early as the first trimester [23]. Not all early discordant twins are anomalous, however, as a recent study of a sample of 16 apparently normal pregnancies found that twins who are ultimately discordant at birth may exhibit differences in growth as early as 11 to 14 weeks' gestation [24].

A second point refers to the association between placental chorionicity and discordance and the significance of this association. A recent study attempted to quantify the incidence of neurologic morbidity in preterm monochorionic and dichorionic twins by the presence and absence of discordance (>20%) [25]. Monochorionic infants had a significantly higher incidence of cerebral palsy and neurologic morbidity than dichorionic infants, and the cerebral palsy risk was higher in infants with discordant birth weight than infants with chronic twin-twin transfusion. Similarly, discordant dichorionic infants had higher neuromorbidity than infants in the concordant group. In discordant infants with both placental types, neurologic morbidity was independent of growth restriction.

Approximately 10% to 15% of monochorionic twins develop twin-twin transfusion, a condition that commonly results in discordant birth weights. When discordant sizes are found in the antenatal evaluation of monochorionic twins, twin-twin transfusion should be excluded. It is recognized that monochorionic twins weigh less than twins from dichorionic gestations after correcting for gestational age [26]. Umbilical cord velamentous insertion seems to be associated with reduced birth weight in all types of twins [27]. It also seems that differences between the mean birth weights of dizygotic, monozygotic dichorionic, and monozygotic monochorionic infants may originate from fused placentas with a peripheral cord insertion, which occurs most frequently in monozygotic twins [27]. Most authors agree that monochorionic twins are more likely to exhibit absolute growth restriction and low birth weight. The question of whether monochorionic twins also exhibit discordant growth remains controversial, however, with reports showing a more than twofold likelihood of severe discordance among monochorionic twins [28,29] and reports finding similar discordance frequencies in the two placental types [30–33]. Although the likelihood of having one or two small-for-gestational-age twins has not been explored extensively by placental type [28,32], it seems that intrauterine growth restriction—but not discordance—is more frequent among monochorionic twins.

The third and final point is the use of ancillary signs of fetal well-being when growth aberrations are suspected. It is logical that methods suitable for singletons are also suitable for twins or higher-order multiples. For example, the biophysical profile used in singletons is also useful for assessing multiples; however, it is sometimes not easy to quantify the amniotic fluid index in each of the sacs [34] or elicit an interpretable dual fetal heart rate tracing [35,36].

It was expected that Doppler velocimetry of the umbilical [37] and uterine arteries [38] would enhance the sonographic diagnosis of twin discordance [37] and improve outcomes of multiple pregnancies. The sensitivity of abnormal uterine artery Doppler results defined by singleton standards was 9.7% for intrauterine growth restriction, 7.9% for birth weight discordance of 20% or more, and 10.3% for any adverse outcome [38]. The authors of this study concluded that despite using specially constructed twin nomograms, uterine artery Doppler studies in twin gestations had an overall low sensitivity in predicting adverse obstetric outcome. More recently, Giles et al [39] reported the results of a prospective, randomized, controlled multicenter trial of women with twin pregnancies who were randomized at 25 weeks' gestation to receive either standard ultrasound biometric assessment or standard assessment plus Doppler ultrasound umbilical artery flow velocity waveform analysis. Sonography was repeated at 30 and 35 weeks' gestation unless otherwise indicated. The authors did not find a significant difference in the perinatal mortality rate in the no-Doppler group (11/1000 live births) versus the Doppler group (9/1000 live births). The three unexplained intrauterine deaths in the no-Doppler group were considered unlikely to be influenced by Doppler surveillance. In this study, close surveillance in twin pregnancy resulted in a lower-than-expected fetal mortality rate from 25 weeks' gestation in the no-Doppler and Doppler groups, but Doppler evaluation did not seem to add any advantage [39].

Although the concept of physiologic adaptive mechanisms underlying growth aberrations in multiples seems plausible in many instances, not all small multiples are normally grown. On the contrary, adaptation may fail when the uterine milieu is exhausted, manifested by the onset of pathologic events such as placental insufficiency [11,12]. Sonography, despite its limited accuracy to detect birth weight discordance, remains the best (and only) means of following growth patterns of the individual multiple fetuses. A bi-weekly sonographic scan, starting at 28 weeks' gestation, may identify a changing growth pattern, regardless of the growth curves used. Reference should be made to the absolute value shown in various charts for twins and triplets when growth restriction is suspected [3].

Whenever an SGA fetus is observed in a multiple pregnancy, it should be treated in an unprejudiced manner: the pregnancy should be followed as any other pregnancy with an SGA fetus. The size of the smaller twin also should be used to determine if the entire gestation is with or without excess risk of perinatal mortality [9]. This algorithm might reduce many unnecessary iatrogenic preterm multiple births [10,40].

As a note of caution, it should be remembered that none of the management protocols for growth aberration among twins was examined by a randomized, controlled trial. Retrospective data—even population-based registries—do not truly represent the natural frequencies of growth aberrations, because frequencies may be entirely skewed because of preterm deliveries indicated, wrongly or not, for these reasons. The cited frequencies might represent better the effect of the policy of intervention on natural growth pattern of multiples [4]. Because the maternal-fetal and feto-fetal relationships in a multiple pregnancy are exceedingly complex, numerous confounders influencing growth that need careful consideration are inadvertently introduced. An incomplete list of confounders may include parity [5,8,18,19], fetal gender [41], and maternal phenotypic characteristics [20,42].

As a final statement, it should be stressed that the key in management of multiples might lie in the ability to recognize the transition from the physiologic adaptation to the pathologic process of growth restriction.

Patient counseling

When a patient is diagnosed with multiples during the first antenatal visit, she may wish to know her a-priori chance of having very or extremely low birth weight infants and how is it possible to reduce the odds of having low birth weight multiples. In twins, the overall risk of having at least one VLBW (< 1500 g) infant was 1:5 among nulliparas and 1:12 among multiparas [43]. The risk of having two VLBW twins among nulliparas (1:11) was double that of multiparas (1:22).

In triplets, the odds of delivering at least one extremely low birth weight (< 1000 g) infant also was significantly higher among nulliparas (1:8) than among multiparas (1:14), and the odds of having at least two extremely low birth weight siblings in nulliparas (1:16) is twice higher than in multiparas (1:31). Nulliparas and multiparas, however, have statistically similar odds of delivering three extremely low birth weight infants (1:29 versus 1:40) [44].

The difference between nulliparas and multiparas is not the only one that may influence the chance of the expecting mother of multiples for an adverse outcome in terms of birth weight. For instance, maternal age, especially after age 40, seems to improve these outcomes in triplets [45], as does maternal stature [20,42]. Recently, a score that comprised pregravid maternal characteristics was constructed; it assigned one point for the presence of a risk factor (eg, nulliparity, stature < 165 cm, and age < 35 years) and zero for the absence of a risk factor [42]. In 18% of triplets' mothers with a score of 3, the likelihood for adverse results (total triplet birth weight < 4500 and delivery at 27–32 weeks' gestation) was 50% to 90% higher, and the likelihood for optimal results (total triplet birth weight > 6000 g and delivery at > 33 weeks' gestation) was 40% to 70% lower than background rates [42]. These data suggest that a pregravid maternal profile could estimate the likelihood of adverse outcomes and be used for consulting patients at risk of having or carrying a triplet pregnancy.

Because the previously mentioned maternal characteristics cannot be changed, the only available remedy to improve outcomes in terms of birth weight emerges from nutritional intervention pioneered by Luke and co-workers. Luke et al [46] reported that maternal weight gain early during pregnancy might improve outcomes of twins and triplets [47]. This conclusion is based on the underlying common sense that in multiples, a greater need to provide for more "fetal" mass exists earlier in pregnancy. When appropriately met by adequate maternal weight gain, improved outcomes are expected in terms of prolonging length of gestation and in larger birth weights [46,47]. Our group (Sharma et al, unpublished observation) recently confirmed that above-average weight gain during the first 24 weeks of triplet gestations improved neonatal outcomes in terms of greater total triplet birth weights and less frequent VLBW neonates in nulliparas and multiparas. The recommended weight gain in relation to potential confounders, such as parity and prepregnancy body mass index, must be further studied in large series [48].

Summary

Growth of twins and higher-order multiples is an exceptional metabolic challenge for the expecting mother. She is doing much more than a mother of a singleton in terms of nurturing, however. These metabolic requirements need adequate dietary intervention in the form of increased weight gain during early pregnancy.

Regardless of any intervention, the uterine milieu is limited in its ability to nurture multiples in the human female; therefore, it is normal for multiples to be smaller than singletons. Being smaller than singletons does not necessarily mean that multiples are pathologically growth restricted. It is important to remember that twins and triplets have different growth patterns, and their growth should not be considered by using singleton standards. Twins and triplets are not two or three singletons that just happen to convene at the same time and at the same place.

When an SGA fetus is suspected in a multiple pregnancy, it is advisable to follow or to treat the pregnancy as if it was an SGA singleton. Intervention should follow the same guidelines as for singletons.

References

[1] Martin JA, Hamilton BE, Sutton PD, et al. Births: final data for 2002. Natl Vital Stat Rep 2003;52:1–113.
[2] Alexander GR, Kogan M, Martin J, et al. What are the fetal growth patterns of singletons, twins, and triplets in the United States? Clin Obstet Gynecol 1998;41:114–25.
[3] Blickstein I. Is it normal for multiples to be smaller than singletons? Best Pract Res Clin Obstet Gynaecol 2004;18:613–23.
[4] Blickstein I, Kalish RB. Birth weight discordance in multiple pregnancy. Twin Res 2003;6: 526–31.
[5] Blickstein I, Jacques DL, Keith LG. Total and individual triplet birth weigh as a function of gestational age. Am J Obstet Gynecol 2002;186:1372–5.
[6] Blickstein I, Kalish RB, Sharma G, et al. The ponderal index in triplets: I. Relationship to small for gestational age neonates. J Perinat Med 2004;32:62–5.
[7] Blickstein I, Shoham-Schwartz Z, Lancet M, et al. Characterization of the growth-discordant twin. Obstet Gynecol 1987;70:11–5.
[8] Blickstein I, Goldman RD, Smith-Levitin M, et al. The relation between inter-twin birth weight discordance and total twin birth weight. Obstet Gynecol 1999;93:113–6.
[9] Blickstein I, Keith LG. Neonatal mortality rates among growth discordant twins, classified according to the birth weight of the smaller twin. Am J Obstet Gynecol 2004;190:170–4.
[10] Hollier LM, McIntire DD, Leveno KJ. Outcome of twin pregnancies according to intrapair birth weight differences. Obstet Gynecol 1999;94:1006–10.
[11] Demissie K, Ananth CV, Martin J, et al. Fetal and neonatal mortality among twin gestations in the United States: the role of intrapair birth weight discordance. Obstet Gynecol 2002; 100:474–80.
[12] Branum AM, Schoendorf KC. The effect of birth weight discordance on twin neonatal mortality. Obstet Gynecol 2003;101:570–4.
[13] Jones JS, Newman RB, Miller MC. Cross-sectional analysis of triplet birth weight. Am J Obstet Gynecol 1991;164:135–40.
[14] Mordel N, Benshushan A, Zajicek G, et al. Discordancy in triplets. Am J Perinatol 1993;10: 224–5.
[15] Fountain SA, Morrison JJ, Smith SK, et al. Ultrasonographic growth measurements in triplet pregnancies. J Perinat Med 1995;23:257–63.
[16] Blickstein I, Jacques DL, Keith LG. A novel approach to intertriplet birth weight discordance. Am J Obstet Gynecol 2003;188:172–6.
[17] Jacobs AR, Demissie K, Jain NJ, et al. Birth weight discordance and adverse fetal and neonatal outcomes among triplets in the United States. Obstet Gynecol 2003;101:909–14.

[18] Blickstein I, Goldman RD, Mazkereth R. Adaptive growth restriction as a pattern of birth weight discordance in twin gestations. Obstet Gynecol 2000;96:986–90.

[19] Blickstein I, Goldman RD. Intertwin birth weight discordance as a potential adaptive measure to promote gestational age. J Reprod Med 2003;48:449–54.

[20] Blickstein I, Jacques DL, Keith LG. Effect of maternal height on gestational age and birth weight in nulliparous mothers of triplets with a normal pregravid body mass index. J Reprod Med 2003;48:335–8.

[21] Blickstein I, Manor M, Levi R, et al. Is intertwin birth weight discordance predictable? Gynecol Obstet Invest 1996;42(2):105–8.

[22] Caravello JW, Chauhan SP, Morrison JC, et al. Sonographic examination does not predict twin growth discordance accurately. Obstet Gynecol 1997;89(4):529–33.

[23] Weissman A, Achiron R, Lipitz S, et al. The first-trimester growth-discordant twin: an ominous prenatal finding. Obstet Gynecol 1994;84:110–4.

[24] Kalish RB, Chasen ST, Gupta M, et al. First trimester prediction of growth discordance in twin gestations. Am J Obstet Gynecol 2003;189:706–9.

[25] Adegbite AL, Castille S, Ward S, et al. Neuromorbidity in preterm twins in relation to chorionicity and discordant birth weight. Am J Obstet Gynecol 2004;190:156–63.

[26] Ananth CV, Vintzileos AM, Shen-Schwarz S, et al. Standards of birth weight in twin gestations stratified by placental chorionicity. Obstet Gynecol 1998;91(6):917–24.

[27] Loos RJ, Derom C, Derom R, et al. Birthweight in liveborn twins: the influence of the umbilical cord insertion and fusion of placentas. Br J Obstet Gynaecol 2001;108:943–8.

[28] Victoria A, Mora G, Arias F. Perinatal outcome, placental pathology, and severity of discordance in monochorionic and dichorionic twins. Obstet Gynecol 2001;97:310–5.

[29] Gonzalez-Quintero VH, Luke B, O'Sullivan MJ, et al. Antenatal factors associated with significant birth weight discordancy in twin gestations. Am J Obstet Gynecol 2003;189:813–7.

[30] Dube J, Dodds L, Armson BA. Does chorionicity or zygosity predict adverse perinatal outcomes in twins? Am J Obstet Gynecol 2002;186:579–83.

[31] Snijder MJ, Wladimiroff JW. Fetal biometry and outcome in monochorionic vs. dichorionic twin pregnancies: a retrospective cross-sectional matched-control study. Ultrasound Med Biol 1998;24:197–201.

[32] Sebire NJ, D'Ercole C, Soares W, et al. Intertwin disparity in fetal size in monochorionic and dichorionic pregnancies. Obstet Gynecol 1998;91:82–5.

[33] Hanley ML, Ananth CV, Shen-Schwarz S, et al. Placental cord insertion and birth weight discordancy in twin gestations. Obstet Gynecol 2002;99:477–82.

[34] Magann EF, Chauhan SP, Whitworth NS, et al. Determination of amniotic fluid volume in twin pregnancies: ultrasonographic evaluation versus operator estimation. Am J Obstet Gynecol 2000;182:1606–9.

[35] Gallagher MW, Costigan K, Johnson TR. Fetal heart rate accelerations, fetal movement, and fetal behavior patterns in twin gestations. Am J Obstet Gynecol 1992;167:1140–4.

[36] Bernardes J, Costa-Pereira A, Calejo L, et al. Fetal heart rate baselines in twins: interobserver agreement in antepartum estimation. Reprod Med 2000;45:105–8.

[37] Sherer DM, Divon MY. Fetal growth in multifetal gestation. Clin Obstet Gynecol 1997;40:764–70.

[38] Geipel A, Berg C, Germer U, et al. Doppler assessment of the uterine circulation in the second trimester in twin pregnancies: prediction of pre-eclampsia, fetal growth restriction and birth weight discordance. Ultrasound Obstet Gynecol 2002;20:541–5.

[39] Giles W, Bisits A, O'Callaghan S, et al, and the DAMP Study Group. The Doppler assessment in multiple pregnancy randomised controlled trial of ultrasound biometry versus umbilical artery Doppler ultrasound and biometry in twin pregnancy. Br J Obstet Gynaecol 2003;110:593–7.

[40] Talbot GT, Goldstein RF, Nesbitt T, et al. Is size discordancy an indication for delivery of preterm twins? Am J Obstet Gynecol 1997;177:1050–4.

[41] Goldman R, Blumrozen E, Blickstein I. The influence of a male twin on birth weight of its female co-twin: a population-based study. Twin Res 2003;6:173–6.

[42] Blickstein I, Rhea DJ, Keith LG. The likelihood of adverse outcomes in triplet pregnancies estimated by pregravid maternal characteristics. Fertil Steril 2004;81:1079–82.

[43] Blickstein I, Goldman RD, Mazkereth R. Risk for one or two very low birth weight twins: a population study. Obstet Gynecol 2000;96:400–2.

[44] Blickstein I, Jacques DL, Keith LG. The odds of delivering one, two or three extremely low birth weight (<1000 g) triplet infants: a study of 3288 sets. J Perinat Med 2002;30:359–63.

[45] Keith LG, Goldman RD, Breborowicz G, et al. Triplet pregnancies in mothers age 40 or older: a matched control study. J Reprod Med 2004;49:683–8.

[46] Luke B, Min S-J, Gillespie B, et al. The importance of early weight gain in the intrauterine growth and birth weight of twins. Am J Obstet Gynecol 1998;179:1155–61.

[47] Luke B. Maternal nutrition. In: Newman RB, Luke B, editors. Multifetal pregnancy. Philadelphia: Lippincott Williams and Wilkins; 2000. p. 192–219.

[48] Nugent LB, van de Van C, Martin D, et al. The association between maternal factors and perinatal outcomes in triplet pregnancies. Am J Obstet Gynecol 2002;187:752–7.

ELSEVIER
SAUNDERS

Obstet Gynecol Clin N Am
32 (2005) 55–67

OBSTETRICS AND
GYNECOLOGY
CLINICS
OF NORTH AMERICA

Risk of Cerebral Palsy in Multiple Pregnancies

Peter O.D. Pharoah, MD, MSc, FRCP, FRCPCH, FFPHM

*Department of Public Health, FSID Unit of Perinatal and Paediatric Epidemiology,
Muspratt Building, University of Liverpool, Liverpool L69 3GB, United Kingdom*

It is pertinent to appreciate that when considering the risk of cerebral palsy (CP) in multiple pregnancies, the syndrome is not a single nosologic entity and various pathologic processes may give rise to the clinical features of the syndrome. Some of the risk factors associated with these pathologic processes occur more commonly in multiple than in singleton pregnancies. Some risk factors may be peculiar to multiple pregnancies, however, particularly monochorionic (MC) and monozygotic (MZ) multiple pregnancies.

The article by Little [1] with the earliest clinical description of CP in 1862 was entitled "On the incidence of abnormal parturition, difficult labor, premature birth and asphyxia neonatorum on the mental and physical condition of the child, especially in relation to deformities." Inherent in the title are risk factors that are more prevalent in multiple than singleton pregnancies.

For many years, peripartum birth injury or hypoxic-ischemic cerebral impairments were considered to be the main cause of CP. This presumed cause was appealing because it was considered that with improved obstetric and neonatal care, early detection of fetal distress, and pre-emptive induction of labor or Caesarean section, there would be a significant reduction in the prevalence of CP. These hopes were not fulfilled, and although perinatal mortality rates fell significantly, there was no concurrent decline in CP rates among term infants [2]. Some studies reported an increase in the prevalence among very low birth weight infants [3–5], which led to a reappraisal of possible causes of CP [6–9].

The timing of the insult that leads to CP may be conveniently divided into prepartum, peripartum, and postnatal periods. CP sustained from a postnatal

E-mail address: p.o.d.pharoah@liverpool.ac.uk

doi:10.1016/j.ogc.2004.10.002
obgyn.theclinics.com

insult also has been termed acquired [10–12] or late impairment CP [13]. This group comprises approximately 10% of all cases of CP [14,15], and the major causes are head injury, cerebral infections, hypoxia, and gastroenteritis with severe dehydration. Multiple compared with singleton gestations are not especially at risk in this category of CP and are not considered further.

At one time, peripartum sustained cerebral impairment as a result of birth asphyxia was considered to be most frequent cause of CP. The failure of CP prevalence to decrease with falling perinatal mortality rates [2], the lack of association of CP with indicators of birth asphyxia [16], and poor obstetric care and the positive association with adverse antenatal events [17] have relegated birth asphyxia to a minor role. Undoubtedly, severe birth asphyxia may cause CP. Studies based on the National Collaborative Perinatal Project and the Western Australian CP register estimated that 3% to 13% and 8%, respectively, of CP was attributable to birth asphyxia [16,18]. In estimating what proportion of CP may be attributable to birth asphyxia, the problems lie in the defining criteria and the fact that these criteria, such as markers of fetal distress and low Apgar scores, may be the result rather than the cause of CP.

Multiple compared with singleton gestations are not at especially increased risk of birth asphyxial events that result in CP. These events, together with postnatal causes, account for approximately 20% of all cases of CP. This leaves approximately 80% of CP that is sustained prepartum or as a result of hypoxic-ischemic damage attributable to difficulties in maintaining physiologic normality in blood pressure and oxygenation in extremely preterm infants. The important role played by prepartum risk factors is supported by the observation that a high proportion of children with CP showed intrauterine growth restriction [19,20] and a higher proportion of coincident congenital anomalies and other dysmorphic features than controls [16]. In this group, clinically important and etiologically significant differences are found between singleton and multiple births, which is the focus of the rest of this article.

Multiple versus singleton birth differences in crude cerebral palsy prevalence

The greater risk of CP in multiple compared with singleton gestations was recognized by Freud more than a century ago [21]. A review of case series reports found that twins comprised 5% to 10% of CP but only 1.6% of all births [22], which indicated a twin:singleton relative risk of approximately 5. The development of population-based registers of CP has enabled prevalence comparisons to be made for multiple and singleton births. Combined data from two registries [23,24] showed relative risks for twins and triplets compared with singletons to be 4.9 and 12.7, respectively, and a large collaborative report based on five population-based studies found that twins were at a fourfold increased risk of CP compared with twins [25].

Risk factors for cerebral palsy in multiple and singleton gestations

One important risk factor for CP in multiple and singleton births is birth weight, with a sharp rise in prevalence of CP with decreasing birth weight [26]. Combined data from three population-based registries show that the relative risks of CP in birth weight groups of 1000 g, 1000 to 1499 g, and 1500 to 2499 g compared with 2500 g or more are 66.5, 57.4, and 8.9, respectively [27]. The shift to the left in the birth weight frequency distribution of multiple births plays a significant role in the higher prevalence of CP in multiple compared with singleton births. Fig. 1, drawn from 1993 to 2000 national data for England and Wales, shows the birth weight frequency distribution for all live births by multiplicity of birth. To subdivide twins into MZ and DZ groups, Weinberg's rule has been applied [28]. This rule assumes that all unlike sex twin are DZ and that the same number of like-sex twins are DZ. The total number of DZ twins is twice the number of unlike sex twins, and the total number of MZ twins is all twins minus the number of unlike sex pairs.

Infants of birth weight less than 1500 g comprise 0.9% of singleton, 9.4% of twins, 32.2% of triplets, and 73.3% of quadruplet live births [29]. It is pertinent also that the birth weight frequency distribution of MZ twins is shifted to the left of DZ twins. In twins, the lower the birth weight, the greater the proportion that is MZ, and there is a highly significant statistical trend in the association of birth weight with zygosity. In twins of birth weight less than 1500 g, 41% are MZ compared with infants who weigh 2500 g or more, in which 28% are MZ.

Because birth weight is an important confounder, birth weight–specific rather than crude prevalence should be examined when comparing CP prevalence in

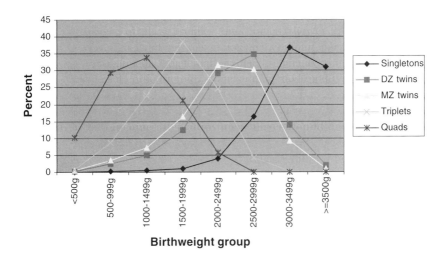

Fig. 1. Birth weight frequency distribution of singletons and multiples.

Table 1
Birth weight–specific prevalence of cerebral palsy in singletons and multiples

Birthweight		Singletons	Twins	Triplets
< 1500g	No. CP	230	56	7
	No. infant survivors	3810	934	179
	CP prevalence/1000	60.4	60.0	39.1
	(95% CI)	(53.2–68.4)	(46.8–77.1)	(19.1–78.5)
1500–2499 g	No. CP	271	58	5
	No. infant survivors	25487	5492	284
	CP prevalence/1000	10.6	10.6	17.6
	(95% CI)	(9.4–12.0)	(8.2–13.6)	(7.5–40.5)
≥ 2500 g	No. CP	849	33	0
	No. infant survivors	569932	6794	40
	CP prevalence/1000	1.5	4.9	0
	(95% CI)	(1.4–1.6)	(3.5–6.8)	

Data from Pharoah POD, Cooke T. Cerebral palsy and multiple births. Arch Dis Child Fetal Neonatal Ed 1996;75:F174–7; Watson L, Stanley F. Report of the Western Australian Cerebral Palsy Register. Perth: TVW Telethon Institute for Child Health Research; 1999. (*Data from* Refs. [23,24].)

singleton and multiple gestations (Table 1). For infants of low birth weight (< 2500 g), there is no significant increase in risk, but for infants of birth weight 2500 g or more there is a highly statistically significant three- to fourfold increase in risk of CP in twins compared with singletons. There are two major components to the difference in crude CP prevalence between multiple and singleton pregnancies: (1) the greater proportion of multiples that is preterm or very low birth weight and (2) some other factor that is peculiar to the process of multiple gestation.

Twinning, zygosity, chorionicity, and cerebral palsy

It has long been recognized that fetal death of a twin is frequently associated with severe morbidity in the surviving co-twin. There are various central nervous system abnormalities, including polymicrogyria [30–33], multicystic encephalopathy or porencephaly [34,35], ventriculomegaly or hydranencephaly [36–38], cortical atrophy [39], and cerebral infarction [40]. Clinically these neurologic pathologies are usually manifest as CP that may vary greatly in its severity, ranging from some minimal limitation of motor function to severe quadriparesis. Not only may the severity of the motor disability vary but also it may be accompanied by a variable degree of learning or cortical visual disability. In almost all these case reports, the common denominator has been that the gestation was MC.

The high risk in the surviving twin whose co-twin died in utero also has been reported in population-based studies of CP. This risk is approximately 1:10 compared with 1:400 of all births [23,41]. Based on an analysis of two national surveys and a regional survey, birth weight–specific CP prevalence when both twins survive or when only one twin survives and the co-twin is a fetal or infant death is shown in Table 2 [42–45]. Because neither zygosity nor chorionicity was recorded, only like- and unlike-sex twins could be compared. Several salient points may be made from this table. When one twin dies in utero, the CP prevalence in the surviving co-twin is high, regardless of birth weight group and is higher in like- than unlike-sex twins (Table 2). When both twins are live births and one dies in infancy, the CP prevalence is even greater than if the twin had died in utero. Low birth weight twins in this group are at particularly high risk and like-sex twins are at greater risk than unlike-sex twins (Table 2). When both twins survive, like-sex twins are at greater risk than unlike-sex twins, particularly among larger infants (Table 2). The combined data (Table 2) confirms that birth weight is an important factor, but twins of like sex are independently at greater risk than those of unlike sex. These data support the observation that monozygosity—and specifically monochorionicity—plays a significant role in the pathogenesis of CP.

The case reports of CP in the surviving twin associated with late fetal death of the co-twin led to the assumption that only late and not early fetal death

Table 2
Birth weight–specific cerebral palsy prevalence in twins

Birth weight	Like sex		Unlike sex	
	Cerebral palsy/number responders	Cerebral palsy prevalence/1000 infant survivors	Cerebral palsy/number responders	Cerebral palsy prevalence/1000 infant survivors
Cerebral palsy in surviving twin of co-twin fetal death[a]				
< 1500 g	15/91	164.8	3/29	103.4
≥ 1500g	20/246	81.3	2/104	19.2
All	35/337	103.9	5/133	37.6
Cerebral palsy in surviving twin of co-twin infant death[b]				
< 1500 g	44/207	212.6	12/87	137.9
≥ 1500g	8/187	42.8	0/75	0
All	52/394	132.0	12/162	74.1
Cerebral palsy: both twins survive infancy[c]				
< 1500 g	52/984	52.8	17/393	43.3
≥ 1500g	54/12037	4.5	13/5841	2.2
All	106/13021	8.1	30/6234	4.8
Combined cerebral palsy birth weight–specific prevalence[d]				
< 1500 g	111/1282	86.6	32/509	62.9
≥ 1500g	82/12470	4.5	15/6020	2.5
All	193/13752	14.0	47/6529	7.2

[a] Like versus unlike sex, Mantel-Haenszel weighted relative risk 2.60 (95% CI 1.06–6.39).
[b] Like versus unlike sex, Mantel-Haenszel weighted relative risk 1.77 (95% CI 1.01–3.25).
[c] Like versus unlike sex, Mantel-Haenszel weighted relative risk 1.29 (95% CI 0.71–2.21).
[d] Like versus unlike sex, Mantel-Haenszel weighted relative risk 1.76 (95% CI 1.29–2.41).
From Keith LG, Blickstein I, editors. Multiple Pregnancy. (Table 3, Chapter 69). Stamford (CT): Thomson Publishing Services; 2005; with permission.

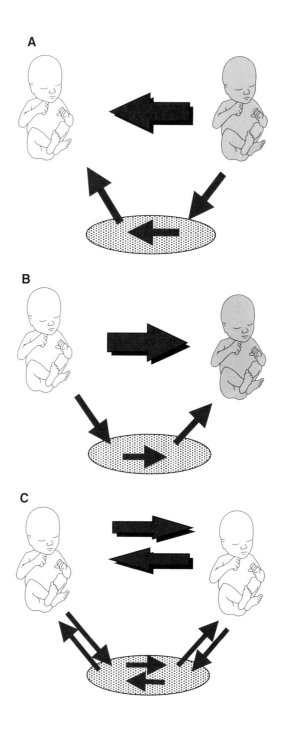

had adverse consequences for the co-twin. This information promulgated the recommendation that early obstetric intervention after fetal death of a twin could prevent neurologic impairment in the co-twin [34], although other researchers questioned the appropriateness of the recommendation [35,46–49]. Subsequently, it became clear that second-trimester demise of a twin also could be complicated by serious morbidity in the co-twin [32,36,40].

The use of ultrasonographic examination in early gestation has established the "vanishing" twin phenomenon, in which first-trimester loss of a twin occurs in 13% to 78% of multiple pregnancies [50]. The prognosis for the surviving twin after such early loss of the co-twin has been considered good, unlike the effect of later fetal death [51]. There have been reports of adverse effects in the surviving twin even after first-trimester loss of the co-twin, however [30,37], and it has been hypothesized that the cause of CP in apparently singleton gestations may be attributable to a vanishing twin [52].

Because monochorionicity is a key feature in the high risk of CP in multiple compared with singleton gestations, early first-trimester recognition of MC gestation with a vanishing twin must be quantified to determine whether it is of etiologic relevance to CP in apparently singleton infants. This determination may require transvaginal rather than transabdominal ultrasound examination soon after conception is recognized. One selected series with a disproportionate number of dichorionic gestations as a result of in vitro fertilization, observed nine MC gestations, of which five delivered twins, one delivered a singleton, and three aborted both fetuses [53]. Although early loss of one twin in an MC gestation is uncommon, it remains tenable that a vanishing twin in an MC gestation could account for some cases of CP.

Also of relevance in pathogenesis of CP in apparently singleton infants is the failure to recognize or register a second-trimester fetal demise that usually presents as a fetus papyraceus. The World Health Organization definition of fetal death is "death before the complete expulsion or extraction from its mother of a product of conception irrespective of the duration of the pregnancy." For countries that subscribe to this definition, the requirement is for a fetus papyraceus to be registered as a stillbirth regardless of the gestational age at which fetal demise occurred. In the United States, the definition promulgated by the World Health Organization but revised in the 1992 Revision of the Model State Vital Statistics Act and Regulations is recommended. The Model State Vital Statistics Act recommends reporting the death of a fetus of 350 g or more or, if weight is unknown, of 20 complete weeks' gestation or more. The implication for a fetus papyraceus varies. It should be reported in all areas that require fetal

Fig. 2. Mechanisms of fetal damage in MC twins. (*A*) Embolic theory: thromboplastin-like material or emboli are transferred through an open placental anastomosis to the survivor. (*B*) Ischemic theory: blood is shunted into the low-resistance circulation of the dead fetus. (*C*) Hemodynamic instability theory: bidirectional shunting leads to ischemic damage that affects either or both fetuses. *From* Keith LG, Blickstein I, editors. Multiple Pregnancy. (Chapter 69, Fig. 1). Stamford (CT): Thomson Publishing Services; 2005; with permission.

deaths to be reported, which would capture a fetus papyraceus because the key feature is the gestational age at delivery and not the presumed gestational age at death. Because not all areas specify how gestational age is calculated, there is variability in interpreting whether the fetus papyraceus should be registered. A similar variability in interpretation exists in the United Kingdom, where the legal responsibility for registering a stillbirth lies with the parents. Obstetricians may not inform a mother that a fetus papyraceus is present so that only the singleton survivor gets registered [54–58]. In a population-based register, of 18 cases of CP in which the obstetric records of the mother had recorded a twin gestation, 6 cases had been registered as only singletons. In all 6 cases, the twin death was a fetus papyraceus or a small, severely macerated fetus of which the mother had not been aware [55].

The variability in the interpretation of the definition of fetal death is surely not confined to the United States and United Kingdom, yet it is of immense significance to the origin of CP and to estimates of the comparative risk of CP in multiple and singleton gestations. Clarification and application of an internationally accepted definition of fetal death are necessary. Registering the presumed gestational age of fetal demise and the gestational age of expulsion regardless of birth weight must be considered.

Pathogenic mechanisms in cerebral palsy

Monochorionicity, with its placental vascular anastomoses, is a common component when there is fetal demise of one twin and CP in the co-twin. Benirschke [59] observed numerous fibrin thrombi occluding blood vessels, which resulted in renal cortical necrosis and cerebral infarction in one case. He proposed that thromboplastin-rich material or thromboemboli were transfused from the dead twin, which led to disseminated intravascular coagulation in the co-twin (Fig. 2A). Although disseminated intravascular coagulation occasionally has been reported after demise of one twin [60–62], it is not always the case, and other pathogenic mechanisms must be considered [36,46,63].

An alternative explanation for the pathogenesis of CP is that the dead fetus has a low vascular resistance with acute twin-twin transfusion and exsanguination of the surviving fetus, which results in ischemic cerebral impairment (Fig. 2B) [64,65].

The mechanisms illustrated in Fig. 2A and B entail fetal demise of one twin. As shown in Table 2, however, there is a high prevalence of CP even when both twins survive. It is particularly notable when both are born alive but one dies in infancy (Table 2). In this group, like-sex twins with a birth weight of 1500 g or more are at risk of CP that is unlikely to be attributable to preterm delivery. Another proposed pathogenic mechanism is that hemodynamic instability with to-and-fro shunting of blood between fetuses may affect either or both fetuses. The severity of damage sustained by the fetuses varies from fetal death to normal survival and may differ between fetuses (Fig. 2C) [66–69]. In these cases, it is the MC placentation per se that lies behind the damage to either or both fetuses.

MC gestations face a double jeopardy for CP. There are problems associated with the twin-twin transfusion effects as a result of placental vascular anastomoses (Fig. 2), and there is a preponderance of preterm infants among MZ compared with DZ gestations (see Fig. 1). A further risk is that the MC subset of MZ gestations is at greatest risk of preterm delivery. The prevalence of birth weight less than the fifth percentile in both twins was 7.5% in MC compared with 1.7% in DC twins [70].

Cerebral palsy and assisted reproductive technology

Inevitably, the rise in incidence of multiple gestations as a result of assisted reproductive technology (ART) has raised concerns over the implication it has for the prevalence of CP [71,72]. Researchers have estimated that there may be approximately an 8% increase in the prevalence of CP in the United States solely because of the increase in multiple births from ART [73]. To the extent that multiple gestations are associated with an increase in prevalence of preterm infants, fetuses conceived with ART—as with spontaneous conceptions—are at increased risk of CP. The extent of MC placentation as a cause of CP in ART gestations is more difficult to estimate. Primarily, ART gestations are DZ and are not at risk because of monochorionicity. Researchers recognize, however, that MZ division occurs more frequently in ART than in spontaneous conceptions. It has been estimated that after artificial induction of ovulation, MZ splitting occurred in 1.2% of cases as compared with 0.45% in spontaneous ovulation, with MZ having occurred in 13 of 126 cases (10.3%) [74]. Among gestations achieved with various ART methods, 7 of 71 (9.9%) were MZ gestations [75]. An analysis of national data that examined the increasing trend in MZ gestations estimated that 15.7% of ART gestations were MZ [76]. The determination of the increased risk of CP in ART gestations ideally requires a large scale follow-up study.

Summary

Multiple compared with singleton gestations are at five- to tenfold increased risk of CP. A major component of the increased risk in CP is associated with the higher proportion of multiple gestation fetuses that are born preterm with cerebral impairment from periventricular hemorrhage or leukomalacia. A greatly increased risk of CP is also associated with MC placentation. It is particularly notable in the surviving twin with fetal or early infant death of the co-twin. The failure to register or record early loss of a vanishing twin or later fetal demise as a fetus papyraceus may lead to a significant underestimate of the risk of CP in multiple gestations and an overestimate of the risk in apparently singleton infants.

The increased risk associated with MC placentation has been variously ascribed to transfer of thromboplastin or thromboemboli from the dead to the surviving fetus, exsanguination of the surviving fetus into the low pressure reservoir of the dead fetus, or hemodynamic instability with bidirectional shunting of blood between the two fetuses. An increased risk of CP in ART gestations is to be expected because of the higher proportion of preterm births. The increase in risk of CP associated with MC placentation will not be observed except for the minority of ART gestations that undergo MZ splitting.

References

[1] Little WJ. On the incidence of abnormal parturition, difficult labour, premature birth and asphyxia neonatorum on the mental and physical condition of the child, especially in relation to deformities. Transactions of the Obstetrical Society of London 1862;3:293–344.

[2] Stanley FJ, Watson L. Trends in perinatal mortality and cerebral palsy in Western Australia 1967 to 1985. BMJ 1992;304:1658–63.

[3] Dowding VM, Barry C. Cerebral palsy: changing patterns of birth weight and gestational age (1976/81). Irish Med J 1988;81:25–9.

[4] Pharoah POD, Cooke T, Cooke RWI, et al. Birth weight specific trends in CP. Arch Dis Child 1990;65:602–6.

[5] Bhushan V, Paneth N, Kiely JL. Impact of improved survival of very low birth weight infants on recent secular changes in the prevalence of cerebral palsy. Pediatrics 1993;91:1094–100.

[6] Illingworth RS. Why blame the obstetrician? BMJ 1979;278:797–801.

[7] Naeye RL, Peters EC, Bartholomew M, et al. Origins of cerebral palsy. Am J Dis Child 1989; 143:1154–61.

[8] Torfs CP, van den Berg B, Oechsli FW, et al. Prenatal and perinatal factors in the etiology of cerebral palsy. J Pediatr 1990;116:615–9.

[9] Bedrick ED. Perinatal asphyxia and cerebral palsy: fact, fiction, or legal prediction? Am J Dis Child 1989;143:1139–40.

[10] Swinyard CA, Swensen J, Greenspan L. An institutional survey of 143 cases of acquired cerebral palsy. Dev Med Child Neurol 1963;5:615–25.

[11] Arens LJ, Molteno CD. A comparative study of postnatally-acquired cerebral palsy in Cape Town. Dev Med Child Neurol 1989;31:246–54.

[12] Pharoah POD, Cooke T, Rosenbloom L. Acquired cerebral palsy. Arch Dis Child 1989; 64:1013–6.

[13] Maudsley G, Hutton JL, Pharoah POD. Causes of death in cerebral palsy: a descriptive study. Arch Dis Child 1999;81:390–4.

[14] Paneth N, Kiely J. The frequency of cerebral palsy: a review of population studies in industrialised nations since 1950. Clinics in Developmental Medicine 1984;87:46–56.

[15] Stanley F, Blair E. Postnatal risk factors in the cerebral palsies. Clinics in Developmental Medicine 1984;87:135–49.

[16] Nelson KB, Ellenberg JH. Antecedents of cerebral palsy: multivariate analysis of risk. N Engl J Med 1986;315:81–6.

[17] Niswander K, Henson G, Elborne D, et al. Adverse outcome of pregnancy and the quality of obstetric care. Lancet 1984;324:827–32.

[18] Blair E, Stanley F. Intrapartum asphyxia: a rare cause of cerebral palsy. J Pediatr 1988;112: 515–9.

[19] Freud S. Infantile cerebrallahumung: Nothnagels specielle pathologie und therapie. [Infantile cerebral paralysis. Translation by Russin LA. Miami: University of Miami Press, 1968.] Vienna: A. Holder; 1897.

[20] Alberman E. Birthweight and length of gestation in cerebral palsy. Dev Med Child Neurol 1964;5:388–94.

[21] Pharoah POD, Cooke T, Rosenbloom L, et al. Effects of birthweight, gestational age and maternal obstetric history on birth prevalence of cerebral palsy. Arch Dis Child 1987;62:1035–40.

[22] Javier LF, Root L, Tassanawipas A, et al. Cerebral palsy in twins. Dev Med Child Neurol 1992;34:1053–63.

[23] Pharoah POD, Cooke T. Cerebral palsy and multiple births. Arch Dis Child Fetal Neonatal Ed 1996;75:F174–7.

[24] Watson L, Stanley F. Report of the Western Australian Cerebral Palsy Register. Perth: Telethon Institute for Child Health Research; 1999.

[25] Scher AI, Petterson B, Blair E, et al. The risk of mortality or cerebral palsy in twins: a collaborative population-based study. Pediatr Res 2002;52:671–81.

[26] Stanley F, Alberman E. Birthweight, gestational age and the cerebral palsies. Clinics in Developmental Medicine 1984;87:57–68.

[27] Pharoah POD, Cooke T, Johnson MA, et al. Epidemiology of cerebral palsy in England and Scotland, 1984–9. Arch Dis Child Fetal Neonatal Ed 1998;79:F21–5.

[28] Weinberg W. Beiträge zur physiologie und pathologie der mehrlingsgeburten beim menschen. Pflugers Arch Gesamte Physiol Menschen Tiere 1902;88:346–430.

[29] Office for National Statistics. Mortality statistics: childhood, infant and perinatal. Series DH3, Nos. 27–33. London: HMSO; 1996–2002.

[30] Baker EM, Khorasgani MG, Gardner-Medwin D, et al. Arthrogryposis multiplex congenita and bilateral parietal polymicrogyria in association with the intrauterine death of a twin. Neuroped 1996;27:54–6.

[31] Bordarier C, Robain O. Microgyric and necrotic cortical lesions in twin fetuses: original cerebral damage consecutive to twinning? Brain Dev 1992;14:174–8.

[32] Van Bogaert P, Donner C, David P, et al. Congenital bilateral perisylvian syndrome in a monozygotic twin with intra-uterine death of the co-twin. Dev Med Child Neurol 1996;38:166–71.

[33] Larroche JC, Girard N, Narcy F, et al. Abnormal cortical plate (polymicrogyria), heterotopias and brain damage in monozygous twins. Biol Neonate 1994;65:343–52.

[34] D'Alton ME, Newton ER, Cetrulo CL. Intrauterine fetal demise in multiple gestation. Acta Genet Med Gemellol 1984;33:43–9.

[35] Fusi L, Gordon H. Twin pregnancy complicated by single intrauterine death: problems and outcome with conservative management. Br J Obstet Gynaecol 1990;97:511–6.

[36] Anderson RL, Golbus MS, Curry CJR, et al. Central nervous system damage and other anomalies in surviving fetus following second trimester antenatal death of co-twin. Prenat Diag 1990;10:513–8.

[37] Hoyme EH, Higginbottom MC, Jones KL. Vascular etiology of disruptive structural defects in monozygotic twins. Pediatrics 1981;67:288–91.

[38] Jung JH, Graham JM, Schultz N, et al. Congenital hydranencephaly/porencephaly due to vascular disruption in monozygotic twins. Pediatrics 1984;73:467–9.

[39] Ishimatsu J, Hori D, Hamada MT, et al. Twin pregnancies complicated by the death of one fetus in the second or third trimester. J Matern Fetal Investig 1994;4:141–5.

[40] Weig SG, Marshall PC, Abroms IF, et al. Patterns of cerebral injury and clinical presentation in the vascular disruptive syndrome of monozygotic twins. Pediatr Neurol 1995;13:279–85.

[41] Grether JK, Nelson KB, Cummins CK. Twinning and cerebral palsy: experience in four Northern Californian counties, births 1983 through 1985. Pediatrics 1993;92:854–8.

[42] Pharoah POD, Adi Y. Consequences of in-utero death in a twin pregnancy. Lancet 2000; 355:1597–602.

[43] Pharoah POD. Cerebral palsy in the surviving twin associated with infant death of the co-twin. Arch Dis Child Fetal Neonatal Ed 2001;84:F111–6.

[44] Pharoah POD, Price TS, Plomin R. Cerebral palsy in twins: a national study. Arch Dis Child Fetal Neonatal Ed 2002;87:F122–4.

[45] Glinianaia SV, Pharoah POD, Wright C, et al. Fetal or infant death in twin pregnancy:

neurodevelopmental consequence for the survivor. Arch Dis Child Fetal Neonatal Ed 2002; 86:F9–15.

[46] Hanna JH, Hill JM. Single intrauterine fetal demise in a multiple gestation. Obstet Gynecol 1984;63:126–30.

[47] Kilby MD, Govind A, O'Brien PMS. Outcome of twin pregnancies complicated by a single intrauterine death: a comparison with viable twin pregnancies. Obstet Gynecol 1994;84:107–9.

[48] Santema JG, Swaak AM, Wallenburg HCS. Expectant management of twin pregnancy with single fetal death. Br J Obstet Gynaecol 1995;102:26–30.

[49] Zorlu CG, Yalçin HR, Çağlar T, et al. Conservative management of twin pregnancies with one dead fetus: is it safe? Acta Obstet Gynecol Scand 1997;76:128–30.

[50] Landy HJ, Keith L, Keith D. The vanishing twin. Acta Genet Med Gemellol 1982;31:179–84.

[51] Landy HJ, Keith LG. The vanishing twin: a review. Hum Reprod Update 1998;4:177–83.

[52] Pharoah POD, Cooke RWI. A hypothesis for the aetiology of spastic cerebral palsy: the vanishing twin. Dev Med Child Neurol 1997;39:292–6.

[53] Benson CB, Doubilet PM, Laks MP. Outcome of twin gestations following sonographic demonstration of two heart beats in the first trimester. Ultrasound Obstet Gynecol 1993;3:343–5.

[54] Heys RF. Selective abortion. BMJ 1996;313:1004.

[55] Pharoah POD, Cooke RWI. Registering a fetus papyraceus. BMJ 1997;314:441–2.

[56] Heys RF. Regulations on registration of a fetus papyraceus need to be revised. BMJ 1997; 314:1352–3.

[57] Griffiths M. Health professionals can exercise discretion. BMJ 1997;314:442.

[58] Gompels MJ, Davies D. Fetus papyraceus is being increasingly registered in Wessex. BMJ 1999;319:1271.

[59] Benirschke K. Twin placenta in perinatal mortality. N Y State J Med 1961;61:1499–508.

[60] Romero R, Duffy TP, Berkowitz RL, et al. Prolongation of a preterm pregnancy complicated by death of a single twin in utero and disseminated intravascular coagulation. N Engl J Med 1984;310:772–4.

[61] Coleman BG, Grumbach K, Arger PH, et al. Twin gestations: monitoring complications and anomalies with US. Radiology 1987;165:449–53.

[62] Skelly H, Marivate M, Norman R, et al. Consumptive coagulopathy following fetal death in a triplet pregnancy. Am J Obstet Gynecol 1982;142:595–6.

[63] Petersen IR, Nyholm HCJ. Multiple pregnancies with single intrauterine demise. Acta Obstet Gynecol Scand 1999;78:202–6.

[64] Golbus MS, Cunningham N, Goldberg JD, et al. Selective termination of multiple gestations. Am J Med Genet 1988;31:339–48.

[65] Fusi L, McParland P, Fisk N, et al. Acute twin-twin transfusion: a possible mechanism for brain-damaged survivors after intrauterine death of a monochorionic twin. Obstet Gynecol 1991;78:517–20.

[66] Bejar R, Vigliocco G, Gramajo H, et al. Antenatal origin of neurologic damage in newborn infants. II. Multiple gestations. Am J Obstet Gynecol 1990;162:1230–6.

[67] Larroche JC, Droulle P, Delezoide AL, et al. Brain damage in monozygous twins. Biol Neonate 1990;57:261–78.

[68] Gonen R. The origin of brain lesions in survivors of twin gestations complicated by fetal death. Am J Obstet Gynecol 1991;161:1897–8.

[69] Grafe MR. Antenatal cerebral necrosis in monochorionic twins. Pediatr Pathol 1993;13:15–9.

[70] Sebire NJ, Snijders RJM, Hughes K, et al. The hidden mortality of monochorionic twin pregnancies. Br J Obstet Gynaecol 1997;104:1203–7.

[71] Imaizumi Y. A comparative study of twinning and triplet rates in 17 countries. Acta Genet Med Gemellol 1998;47:101–14.

[72] Kiely JL, Kiely M. Epidemiological trends in multiple births in the United States, 1971–1998. Twin Res 2001;4:131–3.

[73] Kiely JL, Kiely M, Blickstein I. Contribution in the rise in multiple births to the potential increase in CP [abstract]. Pediatr Res 2000;47:314A.

[74] Derom C, Vlietinck R, Derom R, et al. Increased monozygotic twinning rate after ovulation induction. Lancet 1987;i:1236–8.

[75] Wenstrom KD, Syrop CH, Hammitt DG, et al. Increased risk of monochorionic twinning associated with assisted reproduction. Fertil Steril 1993;60:510–4.

[76] Platt MJ, Marshall A, Pharoah POD. The effects of assisted reproduction on the trends and zygosity of multiple births in England and Wales 1974–99. Twin Res 2001;4:417–21.

ELSEVIER
SAUNDERS

Obstet Gynecol Clin N Am
32 (2005) 69–80

OBSTETRICS AND
GYNECOLOGY
CLINICS
OF NORTH AMERICA

The Paradox of Old Maternal Age in Multiple Pregnancies

Jaroslaw J. Oleszczuk, MD, PhD[a,b],
Louis G. Keith, MD, PhD[b,c],*, Agnieszka K. Oleszczuk, MD[d]

[a]McKinsey & Company, Suite 2900, 21 South Clark Street, Chicago, IL 60603-2900, USA
[b]Center for Study of Multiple Birth, Suite 1015, 680 Lake Shore Drive, Chicago, IL 60611, USA
[c]Northwestern University, Suite 1015, 680 Lake Shore Drive, Chicago, IL 60611, USA
[d]Department of Ophthalmology, Medical Institute of the Department of Defense of the
Republic of Poland, Warsaw, Poland

The demographic patterns relating to births in the United States have changed in the past two decades. Not only are older women giving birth but also older women are having their first birth. Although these facts are undeniable and receive much public attention, little is known about the actual phenomenon of delayed childbearing, possibly because the obstetric literature does not provide a consensus definition of "older gravida." Current definitions are based primarily on arbitrary decision rather than medical evidence, which gives clinicians little guidance at best and completely confuses them at worst. In the past, age 35 was commonly used to separate younger from older parturients. Recent literature most commonly uses 40 years as the threshold, however, although other descriptors are also common (eg, 45 years and menopausal). We do not attempt to unify this definition in this article and use the most common threshold of 40 years to define the "older gravida."

Reasons for delayed childbearing are well known. By far the most important reason is the career-oriented lifestyle that became evident in the last decades of the twentieth century, but other factors are also cited, namely the increasing

* Corresponding author. 333 East Superior, Room 464, Chicago IL 60611.
E-mail address: lgk395@northwestern.edu (L.G. Keith).

0889-8545/05/$ – see front matter © 2005 Elsevier Inc. All rights reserved.
doi:10.1016/j.ogc.2004.10.010

obgyn.theclinics.com

numbers of individuals born to members of the so-called post–World War II baby boom, the increasingly sophisticated armamentarium of fertility control, and late or second marriages. What often is not known—by women or their doctors—is that older age predisposes to high-risk twin or higher-order multiple pregnancies, both as a result of iatrogenic (assisted reproduction) and natural mechanisms. Driven by the lure of assisted reproductive technology, what women and their physicians often overlook is that fertility gradually and inevitably declines from a high at age 20 to 24 to virtually zero at age 45 to 49 regardless of contraceptive use or ethnic status [1]. Little is known about the risks or benefits of delayed childbearing.

The popular view among patients and health care professionals is that older age results in poorer pregnancy and perinatal outcomes. The medical rationale for these observations is twofold. First, the incidence of chronic medical conditions is higher, especially after age 40. Many such women have been infertile or subfertile for many years [2]. Second, regardless of the presence or absence of medical conditions or any degree of infertility, physicians long have tended to consider older gravidas as women who required special attention or special care. The combination of these two factors results in older gravidas being treated differently, regardless of whether there is a scientific basis for such a treatment.

The aim of this article is to review the existing traditional literature on the "older gravida" and present new evidence from multiple gestations that suggests an outcomes paradox: that advanced maternal age may be associated with better outcomes.

Sizing the problem

Tables 1 to 3 show the drastic difference between the age-related birth ratios over time (Table 1), the relatively static rate of live births per 1000 women between 1975 and 1998 at age 20 to 24 compared with the more than 50% increase in women over age 40 (Table 2), and finally, the tenfold increase

Table 1
Maternal age frequencies (per 1 million live births), United States

Maternal age (y)	1971–1977	1990–1992	1997–1998	Ratio 1997–1998/ 1971–1977
20–24	261.8	335.3	432.1	1.7
25–29	394.0	767.9	1376.6	3.5
30–34	413.0	1328.5	2966.5	7.2
35–39	377.5	1690.5	3725.1	9.9
40–44	387.1	799.2	3513.4	9.1
45 or older	461.3	1680.7	23005.9	49.9

Table 2
Live births per 1000 women, 1975–1998, United States

Year	< 20	20–24	25–29	30–34	35–39	≥ 40
1975	56.9	113.0	108.2	52.3	19.5	4.9
1980	54.1	115.1	112.9	61.9	19.8	4.1
1985	52.5	108.3	111.0	69.1	24.0	4.2
1990	61.3	116.5	120.2	80.8	31.7	5.7
1995	58.1	109.8	112.2	82.5	34.3	6.9
1998	52.1	111.2	115.9	87.4	37.4	7.7

in the percent of high-order multiple births in women over age 40 in the last two decades of the twentieth century (Table 3).

"Traditional" evidence from singleton pregnancies

A considerable amount of literature has been published on the outcomes of "elderly" gravidas. Most are concerned with singleton pregnancies and, not surprisingly, they mention higher rates of those conditions with greater prevalence in older women (eg, gestational diabetes, chronic hypertension, the need for cesarean section, hypothyroidism). Three reviews merit particular attention. The first, by Spellacy et al [3], used a computer database of 41,335 women who delivered between 1982 and 1984. Besides corroborating what was found in previous studies, these investigators observed that older women whose weight was less than 67.5 kg (148.5 lb) did not show differences in hypertension, fetal macrosomia, fetal death rates, or low Apgar scores as compared with their younger counterparts.

The second review, by Bianco et al [4], included 1404 pregnant women at least 40 years of age and 6978 controls aged 20 to 29. The two groups were stratified according to parity. Older gravidas were more likely to develop gestational diabetes (nulliparas: Odds Ratio (OR) 2.7, 95% confidence index [CI]: 1.9–3.7; multiparas: OR 3.8, 95% CI 2.7–5.4), pre-eclampsia (nulliparas: OR 1.8, 95% CI 1.3–2.6; multiparas: OR 1.9, 95% CI: 1.2–2.9), and placenta previa (nulliparas: OR 13, 95% CI: 4.8–35; multiparas: OR 6.4, 95% CI: 2.6–15.6). Older women also were at increased risk for cesarean delivery (nulliparas: OR 3.1,

Table 3
Triplets[a] births (% of all births in given year) by maternal age, 1975–1998, United States

Year	≥ 30	≥ 35	≥ 40
1975	25.2	6.4	1.5
1980	29.5	5.5	0.5
1985	34.4	8.6	0.8
1990	54.3	17.4	0.9
1995	66.0	26.5	4.5
1998	70.6	28.6	5.8

[a] Includes triplets, quadruplets, quintuplets, and other higher-order multiples.

95% CI: 2.6–3.7, multiparas: OR 3.3, 95% CI 2.6–4.1), operative vaginal delivery (nulliparas: OR 2.4, 95% CI: 1.9–2.9; multiparas: OR 1.5, 95% CI: 1.2–1.9), and induction of labor (nulliparas: OR 1.5, 95% CI: 1.2–1.8; multiparas: OR 1.4, 95% CI: 1.1–1.7). In contrast, the number of perinatal deaths did not differ by age or parity, and the number of neonatal deaths was too small for comparison. The authors concluded that although maternal morbidity was increased in older gravidas, the overall neonatal outcome was not affected [4].

The largest study on singletons used data from the California Health Information Policy Project that consisted of linked records from birth certificates and hospital discharge records of mothers and neonates that occurred in all civilian hospitals in California from 1992 to 1993 [5]. Approximately 1.16 million women delivered during the study period, and 24,032 (2%) of them were age 40 or older. Of this latter group, 4777 (20%) were nulliparous. The authors found that women aged 40 or over have a higher risk of operative delivery (cesarean, forceps, and vacuum deliveries: 61%) compared with younger nulliparous women (35%). The increase occurred despite lower birth weight and gestational age and may be explained largely by the increase in other complications of pregnancy [5].

Evidence from multiple pregnancies

The only recent study that analyzed outcomes in older gravidas in twin pregnancies was conducted by Blickstein et al [6]. These investigators used a population-based cohort of Israeli twins delivered between 1993 and 1998 to compare birth weight characteristics of 510 and 2102 twin pairs delivered to mothers aged 40 years or older (cases) and 35 to 39 years (controls), respectively. The incidence of twin mothers aged 40 years or older increased 50% during the study period, ten times more than mothers aged 35 to 39. There were significantly more nulliparas ($P < 0.001$, OR 1.54, 95% CI: 1.2–1.9) and more multiparas of four or more ($P < 0.004$, OR 1.38, 95% CI: 1.1–1.7) among older mothers. Regardless of parity, there were no significant differences between mean twin birth weight, total twin birth weight less than 3000 g, 3000 to 4999 g, and 5000 g or more, and frequencies of very low birth weight neonates. The authors concluded that twin births at age 40 or older are significantly more likely among either nulliparas or paras of four or more. They further concluded that birth weight characteristics of twins delivered to older mothers are not different from those delivered to mothers aged 35 to 39 [6].

The outcomes paradox

The interest in the older parturient with multiple gestations accelerated in the past several years, initially as a result of the epidemic of multiples after widespread use of assisted reproductive technology and, more recently, as a result of the publication of two large data sets, one public [7] and one private [8]. Both data sets provided new and unexpected insights into pregnancy and perinatal outcomes with relation to maternal age because they showed outcomes better in older mothers of triplets. Data about older mothers of quadruplets and quintuplets also documented favorable survival outcomes with increasing maternal age [9].

The public data set referred to previously is the Matched Multiple Birth File held by the National Center for Health Statistics of the Centers for Disease Control and Prevention in the United States Department of Health and Human Services [7]. These data consist of all twin and triplet fetal deaths, births, and infant deaths in the United States between 1995 and 1997. A special run of the database was performed by Amy Branum with the following methodology (A. Branum, MSPH, unpublished data, 2002). All complete sets of triplet births with no missing information on gestational age or birth weight were selected initially (n = 5238 sets). Next, only triplet sets with all live born infants (ie, no fetal deaths) were selected (n = 5128). Those triplet sets were then stratified by parity (nulliparous or no previous live births); any sets with missing or inaccurate parity were excluded (n = 465). The final sample size consisted of 4660 triplet sets. In this data set there were 212 mothers aged 40 or older (49 nulliparous and 163 multiparous). For each triplet set born to these mothers, two controls were selected randomly from age group 25 to 29 and 35 to 39 based on same parity (98 nulliparous and 326 multiparous from both of the control age groups). Mean gestational age, total triplet birth weight, individual triplet birth weight, and standard deviations were computed using SAS (v 8.02, SAS Institute, Cary NC, USA).

Neonatal outcomes were found to be better in older mothers (Table 4). Mean gestational age at delivery of mothers aged 40 or older was 33.9 weeks, compared with 32.5 weeks for mothers aged 35 to 39 and 32 weeks for mothers aged 25 to 29. Similarly, the mean total triplet birth weight for mothers aged 40 and older was 5558.5 g, compared with 5153.4 g for mothers aged 35 to 38 and 4951.1 g for mothers aged 25 to 29. At the same time, the mean individual birth weight of triplets born to mothers aged 40 or older was 1852.8 g, compared with 1699.5 g for mothers aged 35 to 39 and 1624.2 g for mothers aged 25 to 29. With regard to multiparous mothers, the mean gestational age at delivery of mothers aged 40 or older was 33 weeks, compared with 32.8 weeks for mothers aged 35 to 39 and 32.2 weeks for mothers aged 25 to 29. Mean total triplet birth weight for mothers aged 40 or older was 5538.9 g, compared with 5399.3 g for mothers aged 35 to 30 and 5069.4 g for mothers aged 25 to 29. Mean individual birth weight of triplets born to mothers aged 40 or older was 1846.3 g, compared with 1799.8 g for mothers aged 35 to 39 and 1689.8 g for mothers aged 25 to 29 (Table 4). The National Center for Health Statistics Matched Multiple Data Set was used further to compare neonatal death rates in complete triplet sets by maternal age. In triplets, the neonatal death rates declined from 54.3 per 1000 in mothers aged 25 to 29 to 21.5 per 1000 in mothers aged 40

Table 4
Results from National Center for Health Statistics matched multiple data file

	25–29		35–39		40+	
	n	Mean ± SD	n	Mean ± SD	n	Mean ± SD
Nulliparous mothers						
Mean gestational age	98	32.0 ± 3.6	98	32.5 ± 3.4	49	33.9 ± 3.6
Mean total triplet birth wt	98	4951.1 ± 1507.3	98	5153.4 ± 1671.8	49	5558.5 ± 1466.3
Mean ind triplet birth wt	294	1624.2 ± 543.6	294	1699.5 ± 596.5	147	1852.8 ± 524.3
Mean ind triplet birth wt						
< 28 wk	27	713.3 ± 299.0	24	594.3 ± 133.0	6	837.7 ± 168.2
28–42 wk	90	1383.6 ± 328.5	66	1307.3 ± 316.4	30	1355.9 ± 226.2
32+ wk	177	1928.9 ± 407.2	204	1982.7 ± 454.5	111	2042.0 ± 436.4
Mean total triplet birth wt						
< 28 wk	9	2139.0 ± 917.0	8	1782.9 ± 391.4	2	2513.0 ± 610.9
28–32 wk	30	4150.8 ± 889.0	22	3922.0 ± 831.9	10	4067.7 ± 412.7
32+ wk	59	5786.8 ± 1010.1	68	59948.3 ± 1148.0	37	6126.0 ± 1162.0
Multiparous mothers						
Mean gestational age	326	32.2 ± 3.8	326	32.8 ± 3.6	163	33.0 ± 3.4
Mean total triplet birth wt	326	5069.4 ± 1638.7	326	5399.3 ± 1596.6	163	5538.9 ± 1570.9
Mean ind triplet birth wt	978	1689.8 ± 584.9	978	1799.8 ± 565.6	489	1846.3 ± 559.7
Mean ind triplet birth wt						
< 28 wk	114	706.3 ± 253.8	69	758.1 ± 233.2	27	645.7 ± 229.8
28–42 wk	225	1634.6 ± 359.1	207	1337.2 ± 335.0	99	1357.8 ± 355.4
32+	639	1979.7 ± 394.0	702	2038.6 ± 425.0	363	2068.9 ± 402.2
Mean total triplet birth wt						
< 28 wk	38	2118.9 ± 694.2	23	2274.4 ± 655.7	9	1937.1 ± 693.7
28–32 wk	75	4093.9 ± 954.5	69	4011.7 ± 876.7	33	4072.6 ± 950.1
32+	213	5939.2 ± 1028.2	234	6115.7 ± 1114.0	121	6206.7 ± 1022.1

Abbreviation: wt, weight.
Courtesy of Amy Branum, MSPH.

or older. In twins, the decline was not as dramatic but was impressive (20.5 per 1000 in mothers aged 25–29 versus 13.2 per 1000 in mothers aged 40 or older) (A. Branum, unpublished data, 2002).

The private data set was analyzed by Keith in 2002 [10,11]. Data were available from a nationwide perinatal database of 3288 live born triplet sets that had been collected between 1988 and 2000 and entered into a computerized system by Matria Health Care, Inc. (Marietta, GA). Consistency of documented information was obtained using internally programmed validation ranges within the system and quarterly audits of randomly selected records. Upon enrollment into the surveillance program, patients gave consent for anonymous data collection for research. Mode of conception was not documented. A matched-for-parity case-control (two controls for each case) methodology was used. A total of 171 triplet sets of mothers aged 40 or older was identified and matched for parity with 342 sets from mothers aged 35 to 39 and 342 further sets of mothers aged 25 to 29. The two-tailed Student t and chi^2 tests were used for continuous and categorical variables, respectively.

Keith concluded the following information based on a case-control study that matched for parity status: (1) mothers older than age 40 had only approximately one third of deliveries at less than 28 weeks versus mothers aged 25 to 29 (2.3% versus 6.4%); (2) mothers older than age 40 had statistically significantly heavier triplets (A, B, and C) versus mothers aged 25 to 29 (P = 0.16; 0.01; and 0.03, respectively); (3) total triplet birth weight was significantly higher for mothers older than age 40 compared with mothers aged 25 to 29 (P = 0.01); and (4) births less than 1000 g were 35% lower in mothers older than age 40 compared with mothers aged 25 to 29 (4.5% versus 7%), whereas births more that 2.5 kg accounted for 9.5% of births in mothers older than age 40 compared with 5.5% in mothers aged 25 to 29 (P = 0.005) [10,11].

In their analysis of quintuplet and quadruplet births in the United States, Salihu et al [9] also concluded that advanced maternal age was associated with better perinatal outcomes. They analyzed 1448 quadruplet and 180 quintuplet births in the National Center for Health Statistics data set. Infants of older mothers (≥35 years old) were compared with those of younger ones (<35 years old) in terms of early mortality indices. Adjusted mortality probabilities were computed by yearly intervals of maternal age. These investigators found that the likelihood for neonatal (OR 2.00, 95% CI: 1.20–3.45), perinatal (OR 2.10, 95% CI: 1.32–3.23), and infant mortality (OR 2.13, 95% CI: 1.28–3.60) were all significantly higher among younger mothers. For each unit decrease in maternal age, the odds of stillbirth, neonatal, perinatal, and infant death increased by 9%, 12%, 13%, and 12%, respectivel,y in a dose-dependent fashion (P for trend < 0.0001).

These conclusions are supported by the study of Blickstein et al, who concluded once again for nulliparas and multiparas (parity controlled) that as maternal age advanced from less than 20 to 40 forty years or more, the number of triplet sets with total birthweights of more than 5000 g increased and the numbers of sets with total birth weights of less than 3000 g decreased (I. Blickstein, MD, unpublished data, 2002) [6].

Further evidence is provided by Salihu et al (H. Salihu, MD, unpublished data, 2003), who in 2003 reanalyzed the National Center for Health Statistics matched multiple data set. Some of their findings are shown in Tables 5–7. Of interest, not all of the age-related differences were statistically significant. When one

Table 5
Gestational age at delivery by maternal age, triplet gestations, 1995–1997

Gestational age at delivery	Maternal age			
	25–29	35–39	40+	P-value
< 28 wk	17.1	9.8	9.1	< 0.0001
28–32 wk	53.2	40.4	40.7	< 0.0001
> 32 wk	46.9	60.2	60.1	< 0.0001

Data from H. Salihu, MD, unpublished data; 2003.

Table 6
Individual and total neonatal birthweight by maternal age, triplet gestations, 1995–1997

Neonatal birthweight	Maternal age			
	25–29	35–39	40+	P-value
Birth weight A (g)	1624.1 ± 14.7	1783 ± 14.1	1793.0 ± 27.9	NS
Birth weight B (g)	1592.6 ± 14.2	1775.7 ± 14.0	1798 ± 29.9	NS
Birth weight C (g)	1558.4 ± 14.1	1723.0 ± 13.9	1737.9 ± 30.1	NS
Mean total triplet birth weights	4880	5376.2	5464	NS

Data from H. Salihu, MD, unpublished data; 2003.

examines the actual differences, however, one could argue that the differences are clinically important, even if not statistically significant.

Zhang et al [12] analyzed perinatal outcomes in women aged 40 and older (using the same National Center for Health Statistics data set) and found that in contrast to the pattern seen in singleton births, twins born to older women are not at greater risk than twins born to younger women and that triplets born to older women actually fare better than triplets born to younger women. They also concluded that the incidence of very preterm births (<32 weeks), very low birth weight (<1500 g), perinatal death, and infant death all progressively declined with increasing age.

Paradox or not: "older gravida" concept revisited

Before conclusions are drawn regarding the paradoxic nature of the previously mentioned findings, one should evaluate critically the available literature on the older gravida. When such an evaluation is undertaken, several missing pieces of evidence are immediately evident: (1) standard definition of what constitutes "older," (2) a consensus of whether older women inherently represent higher or lower obstetric risk, and (3) a clear understanding of whether such pregnancies are associated with an increase in adverse perinatal outcomes. What is also missing is a clear rationale for the observations that have been made.

One important exception to this knowledge deficit is a report by Mansfield and McCool [13]. Because neither author was a physician, these writers were able to approach the concept of "advanced maternal age" from a new perspective.

Table 7
Frequency of neonatal birthweight by maternal age, triplet gestations, 1995–1997

Characteristic (%)	Maternal age			
	25–29	35–39	40+	P-value
<1 kg	19.7	12.7	11.6	NS
1–1.4 kg	16.7	14.4	14.2	NS
1.5–2.5 kg	53.8	60.4	61.5	NS
>2.5 kg	9.8	12.3	12.6	NS

Data from H. Salihu, MD, unpublished data; 2003.

They concluded that prior researchers failed to control for important contextual differences surrounding the pregnancy and childbirth experiences of younger and older women in most studies of advanced maternal age and pregnancy outcomes published until the late 1980s. They further suggested that these contextual differences accounted for a considerable portion of the differential results mistakenly ascribed to reproductive age. They identified three "hidden" factors that affect pregnancy outcome: (1) older women's increasing likelihood of having a chronic disease, (2) altered medical management of pregnancy and labor in older women with resultant iatrogenic complications, and (3) demographic characteristic associated with healthy, middle-class women who postpone pregnancy in contrast to women with either poverty or subfertility. Perhaps more important, the review of the literature failed to show a solid empirical basis for the generally held point of view that middle-age women, especially first-time mothers, were actually high-risk patients. Overall, only 38% of identified studies demonstrated higher pregnancy risk for mature mothers, whereas as few as 28% of the methodologically accurate studies found this result [13].

Not surprisingly, when the same or similar literature was reviewed by two obstetricians, the concept of increased maternal risk with advanced maternal age re-emerged [14]. The authors clearly concluded that "pregnancy after age 40 involves some clearly demonstrable and even unique risks such as decreased fecundity, spontaneous abortion, genetic abnormalities, medical complications, fetal growth abnormalities, dysfunctional labor, cesarean section, and maternal/perinatal death."

In the absences of clear consensus in the literature, scientific due diligence should begin with finding possible explanations to the more controversial findings of better outcomes in older gravidas.

Possible explanations

Are women of advanced age better positioned than their younger counterparts to bear a child? Unfortunately, no direct evidence can be found in the existing literature, which makes life observations and collateral the key source for the upcoming discussion.

Behavioral factors

Older mothers are likely to be more "mature." Many may have finished or be at a solid midpoint in their career aspirations and have the ability or desire to devote 9 months exclusively to pregnancy. Older mothers, especially those who conceived as a result of assisted reproduction, also are likely to have had sufficient time to increase their awareness of the special needs of the unborn fetus. This also means that these mothers are more likely to seek competent obstetric advice early in the first trimester. Because older women may have a higher body mass index and be as weight conscious as their younger counterparts, they may be more likely to eat wisely, obtain a balanced diet, decrease alcohol consumption, and avoid tobacco entirely. Such potential advantages could be associated with a greater likelihood of positive outcomes.

Physiologic factors

Currently, there is no universally accepted explanation for the advantageous outcomes among triplet births in the older gravida. One potential explanation is that prior pregnancy experience influences later outcomes. The cornerstone of this concept lies in the known changes in uterine size that accompany increasing parity. According to Dickinson [15], the nulliparous uterus varies in length from 3.2 to 8.1 cm, whereas the parous uterus varies from 5.7 to 9.4 cm. More important, the weight of the para 0 uterus is 63.2 g compared with 125 g in the para 6 uterus. In contrast, Langlois [16] describes uterine weight in relation to age and parity. His article also presents numerous references that describe further variations in size in addition to those noted by Dickinson [15]. The gravida 0 uterus weight is, on average, 61.1 g, whereas the para 0 uterus weight is, on average, 63.2 g. No separate classification was given for gravida 0, para 0. It is possible that a para 0 woman could be gravida 1 para 0, and the 2 g difference might be related to the effects of a prior pregnancy that ended in an abortion, although its interpretation is speculative. In contrast, the difference between gravida 0 weight (61.1 g) and gravida 6+ weight (124.5 g) is real, as is the difference between para 0 weight (63.2 g) and para 6+ weight (125.7 g) [16]. In both instances, some processes must have happened to the uteri that subsequently were reflected in their physical structure.

In recent years, the complex changes that result from pregnancy-related "organ growth" have been characterized as "remodeling." The molecular mechanisms that initialize and regulate this growth are not well known or understood. In general, it is understood that organ growth involves numerous specific processes, such as cell proliferation, hypertrophy, apoptosis, differentiation, matrix synthesis, and remodeling [17]. According to Lye et al [17], uterine growth is intimately related to specific hormonal changes in pregnancy, including increases in growth factors, such as Insulin-like Growth Factor (IGF)-1 and Epidermal Growth Factor (EGF), both of which induce myocyte proliferation early in pregnancy, thereby creating a "pool" of myometrial cells that subsequently switch from proliferation to hypertrophy under the influence of progesterone and are "remodeled." This physiologic explanation can provide some insight to the findings of Keith (A. Branum, MSPH, unpublished data, 2002). In that data set, 52% of mothers aged 40 or older had a history of abortion compared with 39.6% of the younger control group (aged 25–29). By having abortions, older mothers may have been more likely to possess "remodeled" uteri that were more able to withstand the rigors of distention as the pregnancy progressed. This latter statement is also compatible with the finding that the frequency of uterine irritability among mothers aged 40 or older was lower compared with their younger counterparts (aged 25–29) (40.3% versus 47.1% in Keith's analysis).

If one accepts the concept that the uterus is "remodeled" by the pregnancy experience, one can expect that even a remodeled uterus determines an optimal uterine volume at which its activity is maximal and from the process of "adaptation" cannot proceed further without facing inherent restrictions from overdistention [18]. One of the most commonly circulated explanations in the obstetric literature for the onset of preterm labor in multiple gestations is that the uterus has an inherent upper limit of expansion, after which labor must ensue. This clinical precept does not consider the effect of uterine "remodeling"; however, the increased weight of the uterus based on gravidity, as shown by Langlois [16], is evidence that even pregnancy that ends in abortion results in cell proliferation, which ultimately may affect uterine performance.

It is also possible that prior cell proliferation from the remodeling process may assist in better nourishing the fetuses of older women, just as labor in the multipara is more efficient. This could explain the higher total birth weights of triplets born to older mothers compared with younger mothers.

Zhang et al [12] provided several other explanations for the findings of their study, including the proportion of women using donor eggs and higher proportion of multichorionic pregnancies. They also suggested that the financial resources available to older women might influence pregnancy outcomes. These explanations, however, are circumstantial and do not provide solid, empirical evidence for the observed outcomes.

Summary

The study of multiple gestations in older mothers has been furthered by the analyses of large population-based [2] or quasi–population-based [3] data sets published in recent years. These initial analyses are counterintuitive in that the obstetric and neonatal outcomes of the older mothers (>40 years) are better than those of their younger counterparts (aged 25–29). Currently, it is not clear if older mothers of multiples are advantaged or younger mothers of multiples are disadvantaged. It seems reasonable, however, to conclude that pregnancy after age 40 represents a new obstetric entity, one in which many women will have twins or triplets as a result of assisted reproductive technologies. Despite the generally accepted "truism" that mothers of multiples would fare worse than their younger counterparts, this was not always the case. Younger mothers were found to be at a disadvantage compared with their older counterparts in terms of birth weight characteristics. These findings support the contention that the uterus, unlike the ovary, does not lose its ability to function with age. As a corollary to this statement, it is reasonable to reconsider the likelihood that any prior pregnancy, including one that ended in spontaneous abortion, might affect uterine function in a subsequent pregnancy by providing a better milieu for growth. Further study in this area is clearly warranted, preferably using databases that combine maternal and neonatal data.

References

[1] Stein Z. A woman's age: childbearing and child rearing. Am J Epidemiol 1985;121(3):327–42.

[2] Keith LG, Oleszczuk JJ. Iatrogenic multiple birth, multiple pregnancy and assisted reproductive technologies. Int J Gynaecol Obstet 1999;64:11–25.

[3] Spellacy WN, Miller SJ, Winegar A. Pregnancy after 40 years of age. Obstet Gynecol 1986; 68:452–4.

[4] Bianco A, Stone J, Lynch L, et al. Pregnancy outcome at age 40 and older. Obstet Gynecol 1996;87:917–22.

[5] Gilbert WM, Nesbitt TS, Danielsen B. Childbearing beyond age 40: pregnancy outcome in 24,032 cases. Obstet Gynecol 1999;93:9–14.

[6] Blickstein I, Goldman R, Mazkereth R. Maternal age and birth weight characteristics of twins born to nulliparous mothers: a population study. Twin Res 2001;4:1–3.

[7] Martin J, Curtin S, Saulnier M, et al. Development of the matched multiple birth file. In: 1995–1997 matched multiple birth dataset. NCHS CD-ROM series 21, no 12. Hyattsville (MD): National Center for Health Statistics; 2000.

[8] Blickstein I, Jacques D. The Matria triplet database: 1988–2000. In: Keith LG, Blickstein I, editors. Triplet pregnancies and their consequences. London: Parthenon Publishing Group; 2002. p. 267–91.

[9] Salihu HM, Aliyu MH, Kirby RS, et al. Effect of advanced maternal age on early mortality among quadruplets and quintuplets. Am J Obstet Gynecol 2004;190:383–8.

[10] Keith L. Triplet pregnancies in women over 40 years of age [doctoral thesis]. Poznan, Poland: 2002.

[11] Keith L, Goldman R, Breborowicz G, et al. Triplet pregnancies in the mothers age 40 or older: a matched control study. J Reprod Med 2004;49:683–8.

[12] Zhang J, Meikle S, Grainger DA, et al. Multifetal pregnancy in older women and perinatal outcomes. Fertil Steril 2002;78:562–8.

[13] Mansfield PK, McCool W. Toward a better understanding of the "advanced maternal age" factor. Health Care Women Int 1989;10:395–415.

[14] O'Reilly-Green C, Cohen WR. Pregnancy in women aged 40 and older. Obstet Gynecol Clin North Am 1993;2:313–31.

[15] Dickinson RL. Human sexual anatomy. Baltimore: Williams & Wilkins; 1949. p. 20–2.

[16] Langlois LP. The size of the normal uterus. J Reprod Med 1970;4:220–8.

[17] Lye SJ, Mitchel J, Nashman N, et al. Role of mechanical signals in the onset of term and preterm labor. In: Smith R, editor. The endocrinology of parturition: basic science and clinical application. Frontiers of hormonal research. Basel: Karger Publishers; 2001. p. 165–78.

[18] Csapo AI, Jaffin H, Kerenyi T, et al. Volume and activity of the pregnant human uterus. J Obstet Gynecol 1963;85:819–35.

ELSEVIER
SAUNDERS

Obstet Gynecol Clin N Am
32 (2005) 81–96

OBSTETRICS AND
GYNECOLOGY
CLINICS
OF NORTH AMERICA

Down Syndrome Screening in Multiple Pregnancies

Alexandra Matias, MD, PhD[a],*,
Nuno Montenegro, MD, PhD[a], Isaac Blickstein, MD[b]

[a]*Department of Obstetrics and Gynecology, Faculty of Medicine, Porto,
University Hospital of S. João, Porto, Portugal*
[b]*Kaplan Medical Center, 76100 Rehovot, Israel*

Screening versus diagnosis

Our responsibility as health care givers is to provide parents with accurate assessment of risks rather than create arbitrary definitions of high and low risk. Thanks to screening, which comprises a methodical search, for individuals in an apparently normal population who are at a particular high risk for suffering from a defined pathologic condition, we can offer them a complementary evaluation or a direct preventive/curative measure.

The decision to screen low-risk populations requires a series of prerequisites to make it useful and effective:

- The natural history of the disease should be well known
- The disease should be significantly prevalent
- The test should have a low false-positive rate (high specificity)
- The test should have a low false-negative rate (high sensitivity)
- The test should be simple, safe, reproducible, and reliable
- Benefits should outweigh the risks
- The test should be cost effective

* Corresponding author.
E-mail address: almatias@mail.telepac.pt (A. Matias).

obgyn.theclinics.com

- The test should have equal access to the whole population, regardless of financial status
- The test should be acceptable clinically, socially, and ethically

The aims of screening include an opportunity to communicate with the parents. Parents require explicit and reliable information for an understanding of a normal result and the offered options when screening results are positive. Demographic changes, including pregnancies at older ages and smaller family size, have led to enhanced demand for aneuploidy screening. Older women are more likely to abort and have reduced fertility and, consequently, noninvasive risk evaluation before invasive karyotyping is of special importance. In contrast, in the younger age group, loss of quality of life as a result of having a severely handicapped child may be considered to be more important. Women at any age may benefit from individual risk evaluation.

When applying a screening method systematically, the collective empirical risk (ie, background risk: maternal age and gestational age) is redefined in a corrected individual risk (which depends on the combination of the results of ultrasound findings and maternal serum biochemical tests performed during the course of pregnancy). Such programs aim to identify a subset of women within the general pregnant population whose pregnancy may be at increased risk of being affected by aneuploidy. Whenever this final risk is increased (ie, the screening test is positive), these women may be offered a suitable diagnostic test. In the case of fetal chromosomal abnormalities, the only method of diagnosis is an invasive test, such as amniocentesis or chorionic villous sampling. Invasive testing implies procedure-related fetal losses on the order of 0.5% to 1%, limited capacity of cytogenetic laboratories, and higher costs.

When confronted with the definite diagnosis, parents must be fully informed to be able to make their decision after careful consideration, including adequate ethical aspects, such as genetic counseling, termination of pregnancy, intrauterine treatment of the affected fetus, maternal transportation to a tertiary center, premature delivery, early and highly specialized postnatal care, and early complementary diagnostic procedures for the need of deciding postnatal management.

What is screening all about?

Down syndrome is the most prevalent autosomic chromosomal abnormality in the human race (birth prevalence of approximately 1:800) and accounts for almost 50% of all aneuploidies. The main impact of Down syndrome is its contribution to mental retardation (8%–33% of IQ < 50%) [1]. In addition to mental handicap, a substantial number of children with trisomy 21 have associated malformations, especially of the heart and the gut. Despite increased medical care, life expectancy of trisomy 21–affected individuals who survive early childhood remains reduced, mainly because of leukemia and early-onset Alzheimer's disease [2].

The most important factor that determines the incidence of trisomy 21 is maternal age. This association was noted by Shuttleworth in 1909 [3], who reported that "It would be fair inference...that more than half of the Mongolian imbeciles are last-born children and that from one-half to one-third of the mothers were at the time of gestation approaching the climacteric period..." In the 1970s and 1980s, several authors calculated population-based incidences for trisomy 21, which demonstrated an exponential increase with maternal age [4]. Other non-disjunctional abnormalities are also related to maternal age [5]. Based on this fact, a simple test was introduced for risk evaluation: a high risk for fetal aneuploidy was considered when maternal age exceeded an arbitrary cut-off. Cut-off levels vary widely among different countries; however, the receiver operating characteristic curve, which gives information on sensitivity and specificity for varying cut-off levels, shows that maternal age alone is a poor predictor of fetal aneuploidies. The risk for any woman aged 35 years or older having a child with trisomy 21 is approximately 1:100 and the risk of having any type of chromosomal abnormality is 1:50. This means that 49 of 50 women are unnecessarily exposed to invasive testing. Depending on maternal age distribution (5% of women in the early 1970s and 15% of women in the beginning of the twenty-first century are aged over 35 years), 50% to 70% of affected children are born to younger women who would be called "screen negative."

Maternal age has been a consistent screening method because it fulfils important criteria for an acceptable screening test. It is inexpensive, is universally available, has no intra- or interobserver variation, is noninvasive, and is understandable by the women screened.

In the late 1980s, a new method of screening was introduced that takes into account not only maternal age but also the concentration of various fetoplacental products in the maternal circulation (biochemical screening). The first report that α-fetoprotein was low in trisomy 21 pregnancies was made by Merkatz et al [6]. Shortly after this, two new markers were described. Human chorionic gonadotropin (hCG) levels were raised [7], and unconjugated estriol levels were low [8] in pregnancies affected by trisomy 21. Combining the maternal serum α-fetoprotein, hCG and unconjugated estriol levels (triple test), up to 61% of trisomy 21 cases could be detected for a fixed 5% false-positive rate [9].

In the 1990s, screening by a combination of maternal age and fetal nuchal translucency (NT) thickness at 11 to 14 weeks' gestation was introduced. This method has been shown to identify about 75% of trisomy 21–affected fetuses for a screen-positive rate of approximately 5% [10,11]. In a fetus with a given crown-rump length, every NT measurement represents a factor that is multiplied by the background risk to calculate a new risk.

More recently, the possibility of combining NT and two biochemical markers between 11 and 14 weeks' gestation (the serum concentration of free β-hCG is approximately 2 Multiples of the Median (MoM) higher than in chromosomally normal fetuses, whereas pregnancy-associated plasma protein-A [PAPP-A] is lower [approximately 0.45 MoM]), provided a detection rate of 90% for a screen-positive rate of 5% [12,13].

Twenty years have evolved, and rules have changed in the screening of trisomy 21 for singleton pregnancies. Detection rates were improved and the invasive testing rate has decreased. Although preliminary, screening for trisomy 21 at 11 to 14 weeks' gestation has made its last steps combining the sonographic markers NT and nasal bone and the biochemical markers of free β-hCG and PAPP-A that could result in a detection rate of approximately 95%, for a false-positive rate of 2% [14].

Twinning process: does it matter?

Twins account for approximately 1% of all pregnancies, with monozygotic twinning occurring in one third of twin pregnancies. The incidence of twin pregnancies is increasing worldwide as a result of increased use of assisted reproductive techniques and ageing of mothers, who after 35 years are three times more likely to conceive twins than women under the age of 20 [15]. This trend has a significant impact on health care, because twin pregnancies are associated with a greater incidence of adverse perinatal outcome than singleton pregnancies [16], twice the risk for structural defects [17,18], and a higher risk for chromosomal abnormalities [19], although for the latter with respect, with trisomy 21 is questionable [20].

Chorionicity rather than zygosity determines several aspects of antenatal management and perinatal outcome. Zygosity refers to the type of conception, whereas chorionicity denotes the type of placentation, depending on the time of splitting of the fertilized ova. All monochorionic twins are monozygotic and, assuming there are twice as many dizygotic as monozygotic twin pregnancies, approximately 80% to 90% of dichorionic twins are dizygotic [19,21]. Meyers et al [22] updated these trisomy 21–calculated risks for twin pregnancies based on age dizygosity rates [22]. The indirect information derived from chorionicity definition roughly can approach zygosity determination.

Because false characterizations can occur in 10% to 12% of cases when second trimester scanning is used to ascertain chorionicity [23,24], the earliest possible diagnosis of monochorionic twinning is highly desirable, although it is seldom achieved in practice. The first step toward prenatal diagnosis and screening in multiple pregnancies is the establishment of zygosity (if possible) and chorionicity (approximately 100% correct chorionic assignment is possible in the first trimester of pregnancy). Same sex and monoplacentation strongly suggest but do not prove monozygosity. Zygosity can be determined only by DNA fingerprinting, however. Prenatally, such testing requires an invasive procedure to sample amniotic fluid (amniocentesis), placental tissue (chorionic villous sampling), or fetal blood (cordocentesis).

In contrast, the concomitant appearance of several sonographic criteria assists in the correct diagnosis of chorionicity, the most determinant factor in terms of perinatal prognosis. The criteria are as follows: (1) one placenta with a paper-thin, reflective hair-like septum without chorion between the two amnions (T sign)

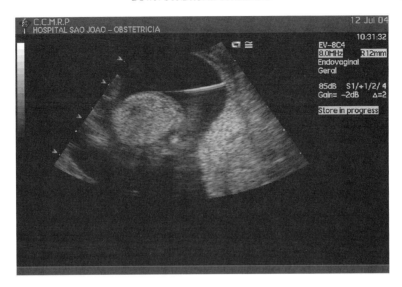

Fig. 1. Example of a monochorionic twin pregnancy at 11 weeks' gestation shows a thin dividing membrane without chorion between the amnion layers.

at 10 to 14 weeks' gestation (Fig. 1), (2) thin septum with less than 2 mm, and (3) same sex in the observed pair.

Conversely, if one finds two separate placentas (Fig. 2) or two fetuses of unlike sex and a lambda or twin-peak sign [25] with chorionic tissue sandwiched between two layers of amnion at 10 to 14 weeks' gestation, dichorionicity is

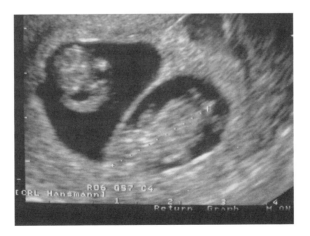

Fig. 2. Lambda sign at 12 weeks' gestation depicts a thick layer of chorion between the two layers of amnion and defines a dichorionic dimaniotic twin pregnancy.

strongly suggested. After 16 weeks' gestation, the lambda sign still indicates dichorionicity [26], but its absence does not exclude dizygosity.

Screening in twin pregnancies

Twins present unique and problematic issues in prenatal diagnosis. The performance of screening tests designed for singleton pregnancies is altered. Surprisingly, recent investigations on this topic are limited despite its increasing importance on daily clinical care.

Screening for chromosomal abnormalities in twin pregnancies raises serious clinical, ethical, and moral problems that must be addressed.

- Effective methods of screening, such as maternal serum biochemistry, are not applicable and have lower detection rates
- In the presence of a "screen-positive" result, no feature suggests which fetus may be affected
- The techniques of invasive testing are more demanding in twins, and there is difficulty in ensuring that fetal tissue is obtained from each fetus
- There is a perceived increased risk of miscarriage with invasive testing in twin pregnancies
- The question is raised as to which invasive test to offer
- There is a paucity of data in abnormally affected pregnancies when the fetuses are either concordant or discordant for an abnormality
- There are difficulties of clinical management of fetal reduction and the potential increased risk to the unaffected co-twin

The overall probability that a multiple gestation contains an aneuploid fetus is directly related to its zygosity. In dizygotic pregnancies, each fetus has an independent risk of aneuploidy, thus, the maternal age-related risk for chromosomal abnormalities for each twin may be the same as in singleton pregnancies, but the chance that at least one fetus is affected by a chromosomal defect is twice as high as in singleton pregnancies. This means that for dizygotic twin pregnancies, the pregnancy-specific risk is calculated by summing the individual risk estimates for each fetus. Because the rate of dizygotic twinning increases with maternal age, the proportion of twin pregnancies with chromosomal defects is higher than in singleton pregnancies.

In monozygotic twins, the risk of an affected fetus approximates the maternal age risk of a singleton pregnancy and, in most cases, the risk for one fetus is, as expected, the same as the risk for the other. This fact ignores the small possibility of heterokaryotypic monozygotic twins resulting from a mitotic non-disjunction after the zygote splits. There are occasional reports of monozygotic twins discordant for abnormalities of autosomes or sex chromosomes, most commonly with one fetus presenting with Turner syndrome and the other being either a normal male or female phenotype, but usually with a mosaic karyotype or Klinefelter syndrome.

The relative proportion of spontaneous dizygotic to monozygotic pregnancies is approximately 2:1, and the prevalence of chromosomal abnormalities affecting at least one fetus in a twin pregnancy would be expected to be approximately 1.6 times that in singletons.

If zygosity is unknown, the risk of at least one aneuploid fetus can be approximated as five thirds that of the singleton risk. This risk is based on the assumption that a third of all twin pairs are monozygotic [19]. Counseling based on chorionicity, clinically more feasible than zygosity, results in the fact that in monochorionic twins both fetuses can be affected equally. If the pregnancy is dichorionic, parents should be counseled that the risk of discordancy for a chromosomal abnormality is approximately twice that in singleton pregnancies, whereas the risk that both fetuses would be affected is a much rarer event, corresponding to the singleton risk squared. With higher risk conditions, such as autosomal recessive disorders, however, this could be as high as 1:16. For example, in a 40-year-old pregnant woman with a risk for trisomy of approximately 1:100 based on maternal age, in a dizygotic twin pregnancy the risk that one fetus would be affected would be 1:50 (1:100 plus 1:100), whereas the risk that both fetuses would be affected is 1:10,000 (1:100 × 1:100). This is, however, an oversimplification, because unlike all monochorionic pregnancies that are always monozygotic, only approximately 90% of dichorionic pregnancies are dizygotic.

When calculating the risk of higher order multiples, estimates can be made by multiplying the singleton risk by the number of fetuses [27]. This method assumes unique chorionicity for each fetus, although monozygosity can occur more frequently than usually thought at higher rates in multiple gestations achieved through assisted reproductive techniques [28,29].

Biochemical screening

Biochemical screening in twins was the first alternative to age-derived risk, but it still can be a source of confusion and has a lower detection rate for fetal aneuploidies and higher rates of false-positive results. In twin pregnancies, the levels of maternal serum markers are, on average, twice as high in unaffected twin pregnancies as in unaffected singleton pregnancies (ie, proportional to the number of fetoplacental units) [20]. When this is taken into account in the mathematical modeling for calculation of risks, it is estimated that serum screening in twins may identify 50% of affected fetuses for a 5% false-positive rate [20].

Another point to consider in biochemical screening is that chorionicity does not seem to affect the distribution and level of maternal serum analytes [30]. Chorionicity does not need to be taken into account when interpreting biochemical markers in twin pregnancies.

In twin pregnancies interpretation of serum analytes is clearly more problematic because each serum marker necessarily relates to the pregnancy and is not specific to the fetus, deriving solely a pregnancy and not a fetus-specific risk.

So far, preliminary studies on maternal serum screening in twins focused on establishing normal values for first- and second-trimester markers [15,30,31]. From a meta-analysis of eight studies regarding the levels of serum analytes in twin gestations in the second trimester [20], researchers have established that the relative median maternal serum levels, compared with singletons, are 2.26 for α-fetoprotein, 2.06 for hCG, and 1.68 for unconjugated estriol. The levels of the screening markers in unaffected singleton pregnancies of the same gestational age can be divided by the twin median levels, and a Down syndrome risk can be calculated by using a singleton algorithm. In this way, a similar false-positive rate presumably could be achieved in singleton and twin pregnancies.

In the first trimester, the same kind of reasoning should be adopted. When considering the calculation of risk in a monochorionic twin pregnancy, in which both fetuses are affected, the median level is simply a multiple of that in an affected singleton pregnancy. For example, the estimated median PAPP-A level in affected monochorionic twins is taken to be 0.80 MoM (1.86 × 0.43), in which 0.43 is the median in affected singleton pregnancies [32] and 1.86 is the median in unaffected twin pregnancies [33]. In affected dichorionic twin pregnancies, it is roughly assumed that the twins are dyzigotic, with one affected and the other unaffected, and that the contributions of the two fetuses to the serum analytes concentration are proportional to the median levels in affected and unaffected singleton pregnancies. For example, the median PAPP-A level in affected dichorionic twins is considered to be 1.33 MoM [((1 + 0.43)/2) × 1.86].

Because biochemical screening in twins is still investigational and far less powerful than in singletons, it should not be recommended in general practice without extensive counseling. Even if prospective studies demonstrate that biochemical screening in twins is effective, several problems must be addressed [34]: (1) The lower detection rate for an acceptable low false-positive rate (altered levels from an affected fetus are, on average, brought closer to the mean and potentially masked by the lower levels of unaffected co-twin, which results in decreased overall sensitivity). (2) If screening is positive, there is no distinctive feature to identify which of the fetuses may be affected. (3) Because serum hCG was significantly increased in twin pregnancies after in vitro fertilization, this fact should be taken into consideration for risk calculation in twins [35]. (4) If the pregnancy is discordant for a chromosomal defect, further management by way of selective termination carries increased risk in the second compared with the first trimester.

Nuchal translucency

The possibility of deriving a risk for trisomy 21 from NT assessment in the first trimester of pregnancy shifted the consideration from a pregnancy-specific risk to a fetus-specific risk. This assumption is based on the observation that the distribution of NT measurements in twin fetuses with trisomy 21 is similar to that in singletons [36–38].

In one of the first studies for trisomy 21 in twins, which involved 448 twin pregnancies, NT was measured in each fetus and the risk was estimated by combining it with maternal age. The NT was above the ninety-fifth percentile for gestational age in 65 of the 896 (7.3%) fetuses, including 88% of those with trisomy 21 [37]. Eight of nine fetuses affected with trisomy 21 were detected, for

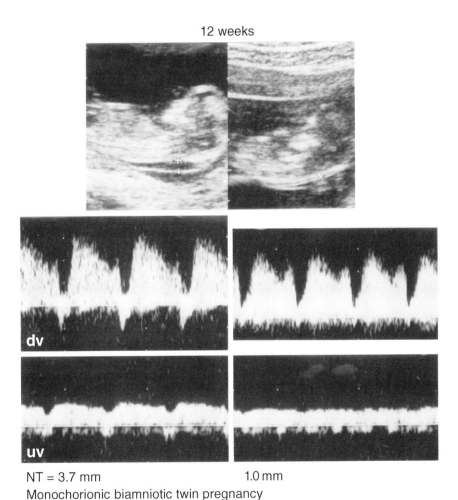

12 weeks

NT = 3.7 mm   1.0 mm
Monochorionic biamniotic twin pregnancy

Fig. 3. A monochorionic biamniotic twin pregnancy was established at 12 weeks' gestation (Case 1). Doppler blood flow waveforms in both fetuses were obtained in the ductus venosus (DV). A discrete NT discrepancy was noted (NT = 3.3/3.7 mm). The fetus with the highest NT shows an inverted A-wave in the DV and later developed signs of TTTS at 18 weeks' gestation.

MATIAS et al

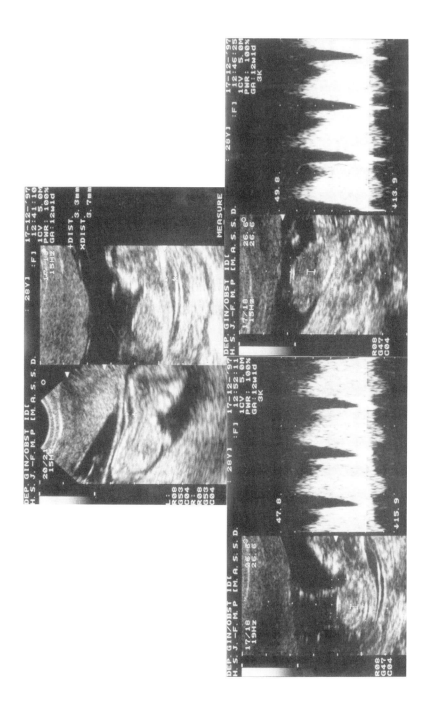

an overall sensitivity rate of 88% which is comparable to the sensitivity rate obtained in singletons. When analyzing the false-positive results, a higher rate was seen in monochorionic gestations (8.4%) compared with dichorionic gestations (5.4%). Increased NT at 10 to 14 weeks' gestation was found twice as much as in monochorionic than in singleton pregnancies, but concomitantly the likelihood ratio of developing twin-to-twin transfusion syndrome in those twins with increased NT was higher (3.5-fold) [16,39,40]. Considering that monochorionic pregnancies do not show a higher prevalence of chromosomal abnormalities, the higher prevalence of increased NT in those twins could be ascribed to cardiac dysfunction. With advancing gestation, this transient heart failure eventually resolves with increased diuresis and ventricular compliance. Later studies by Sebire et al [39] and Spencer [30] found that the NT MoM in unaffected monochorionic twins was not significantly different from the median NT in unaffected singleton fetuses, however. In an ultimate analysis, these data are in good accordance with Sebire's data from 1996 when considering the unaffected monochorionic twins, in which the median NT in those unaffected fetuses is not significantly high (two-tailed chi-squared analysis; $P = 0.119$).

For higher order multiples, the data by which to examine marker distributions in normal pregnancies is even rarer [15,41,42]. More credible data using NT alone to assess risk in triplets or more are described by Maymon et al [43], who attempted to perform trisomy 21 screening in higher order twin pregnancies (three or more) compared with consecutively matched singleton controls. Not only was it feasible and reproducible but also mean NT was similar for both groups (1.41 ± 0.41 mm and 1.35 ± 0.39 mm, respectively, and 0.87 ± 0.23 MoM and 0.83 ± 0.25 mm, respectively) [43].

In a monochorionic twin pregnancy, there is no reason to attribute different risks to the two fetuses, because presumably, both are affected or both are unaffected. It is appropriate to take the average of the two NT measurements to calculate a single risk estimate (averaging method).

In a dichorionic twin pregnancy, the twins are dizygotic in approximately 90% of the cases, which means that one of the fetuses or, much more rarely, both fetuses could be affected. Both fetuses have an independent risk, so it is reasonable to sum the risks on the basis of the NT measurements (summing method). In calculating the risk for each fetus based on its NT measurement and the woman's age, it is necessary to use half the age-related risk, because the background risk of each fetus in a twin pregnancy being affected with Down syn-

Fig. 4. A monochorionic biamniotic twin pregnancy was established at 12 weeks' gestation (Case 3). Doppler blood flow waveforms in both fetuses were obtained in the umbilical vein and DV in the same scan. An NT discrepancy was noted (NT = 3.7/1.0 mm). The fetus with increased NT shows an inverted A-wave in the DV and dicrote pulsatility in the umbilical vein. TTTS developed at 17 weeks' gestation, and the patient was referred for laser ablation of anastomosis. (*From* Matias A, Montenegro N, Areias JC. Anticipating twin-twin transfusion syndrome in monochorionic twin pregnancy. Is there a role for nuchal translucency and ductus venosus blood flow evaluation at 11-14 weeks? Twin Research 2000;3:65–70; with permission.)

drome is, on average, half that of a singleton pregnancy. The 10% of dichorionic twin pregnancies that are monozygotic have their risks calculated incorrectly by the summing rather than the averaging method. The ultimate effect on screening performance is a negligible one, however.

Ductus venosus flowmetry

In recent studies of vascular hemodynamics in fetuses with increased NT at 10 to 14 weeks' gestation, the abnormal flow in the ductus venosus more frequently recorded in fetuses with chromosomopathies, with or without cardiac defects, was related to heart dysfunction [44,45]. These findings are in agreement with the overt hemodynamic alterations found in Twin-to-Twin Transfusion Syndrome (TTTS) later in pregnancy. Accumulated evidence suggests that increased NT along with abnormal flow in the ductus venosus, even in the presence of a normal karyotype, may be early signs of cardiac impairment or defect [40,44,45] (Figs. 3–5).

During a 4-year period, 50 monochorionic diamniotic pregnancies were identified in our ultrasound unit during routine ultrasonographic assessment at 11 to 14 weeks' gestation. NT and Doppler blood flow waveforms in the ductus venosus were recorded in both twins between 11 and 14 weeks' gestation. TTTS was recorded in fetuses that combined increased NT and abnormal flow in the ductus venosus. Until now, in all cases with discrepant NT and abnormal blood flow in the ductus venosus, TTTS eventually developed. In contrast, whenever NTs were discrepant but had normal flow in the ductus venosus, no cases of TTTS were found [46].

Combination of nuchal translucency and biochemical markers for screening of trisomy 21 at 11 to 14 weeks' gestation: the gold standard?

Considering that biochemical screening alone cannot specifically identify the fetus at risk in the presence of twins discrepant for Down syndrome, it seems reasonable to combine NT and maternal biochemical markers, as suggested by Spencer [33]. In this modeled study, the author demonstrated that biochemical screening would add a further 5% to the detection rate obtained by using NT alone and offered a detection rate for Down syndrome of approximately 80% compared with the 90% in singleton pregnancies, which could be a worthwhile addition.

In prospective screening in the first trimester using combined ultrasound and biochemical screening over a 3-year period, Spencer and Nicolaides [47] offered screening to 230 women with twins. The risk for trisomy 21 was calculated for each fetus based on the individual NT and the maternal serum biochemistry corrected for twins. Four cases were observed with twins discordant for trisomy 21, and in 3 cases combined screening identified the affected pregnancy. Of the twin fetuses screened, 6.8% had risks greater than the cut-off, and 9.2% of pregnancies had at least one fetus with an increased risk.

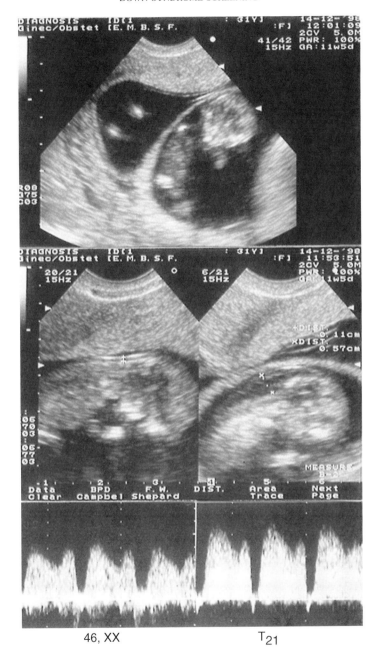

46, XX   T₂₁

Fig. 5. Dichorionic diamniotic twin pregnancy at 11 weeks' and 5 days' gestation. An NT discrepancy (NT = 1.1/5.7 mm) was observed. Doppler blood flow waveforms were obtained in both fetuses. They showed a normal pattern in the fetus with normal NT (46,XX) and a reverse flow during atrial contraction in the fetus with increased NT (trisomy 21).

Table 1
Estimated screening performance in twin pregnancies according to test used and chorionicity and considering maternal age (Adapted from Wald et al, 2003)

Twin pregnancy	Detection rate for a 5% false-positive rate		
	NT (mm) (%)	Combined test[a] (%)	Integrated test[b] (%)
Monochorionic	73	84	93
Dichorionic	68	70	78
All twins[c]	69	72	80
Singletons	73	85	95

[a] NT, free β-hCG, and PAPP-A at 10–13 weeks with maternal age.

[b] NT and PAPP-A at 10–13 weeks and AFP, estriol and free β-hCG, and inibin A at 14–22 weeks with maternal age.

[c] On the basis of the observation that 17% of affected twin pregnancies are monochorionic.

Adapted from Wald NJ, Rish S, Hacksaw AK. Combining nuchal translucency and serum markers in prenatal screening for Down syndrome in twin pregnancies. Prenat Diagn 2003;23:588–92; with permission.

Table 1 shows screening performance in all twins. The estimates are close to those for dichorionic twin pregnancies, because among twin pregnancies with trisomy 21, both fetuses are affected in only approximately 17% of cases. This rate is lower from what could be expected from the observation that approximately one third of twins are monozygotic. The combined test is more discriminative in monochorionic than dichorionic twin pregnancies, because in dichorionic pregnancies the median serum marker level in affected pregnancies is artificially lowered by the unaffected twin, whereas in monochromic pregnancies no dilution of the serum markers is expected from an unaffected pregnancy.

Summary

First or second trimester screening in twin pregnancies is feasible and still efficacious by using either a combination of ultrasound and maternal serum biochemistry in the first trimester (80% detection rate) or maternal serum biochemistry in the second trimester (50%–55% detection rate). These "pseudo-risks" have been challenged for their scientific and clinical validity, however.

Until more data are available from larger studies on the distribution of markers in concordant or discordant twins, NT estimated for each fetus should be the predominant factor by which women who present with increased risk should be counseled regarding invasive testing. In dizygotic pregnancies, pregnancy-specific risk should be calculated by summing the individual risk estimates for each fetus. In monozygotic twins, the risk should be calculated based on the geometric mean of both NT measurements, not forgetting that the false-positive rate of NT screening is expectantly higher than in singletons. The calculated detection rates modeled using this method are still 10% lower than in singleton pregnancies.

References

[1] Hagberg B. Severe mental retardation in Swedish children born 1959–1970: epidemiological panorama and causative factors. Ciba Found Symp 1978;59:29–51.

[2] Yang Q, Rasmussen SA, Friedman JM. Mortality associated with Down's syndrome in the USA from 1983 to 1997: a population-based study. Lancet 2002;359:1019–25.

[3] Shuttleworth GE. Mongolian imbecility. BMJ 1909;2:661–5.

[4] Hook EB. Rates of chromosome abnormalities at different maternal ages. Obstet Gynecol 1981; 58:282–5.

[5] Snijders RJM, Holzgreve W, Cuckle H, et al. Maternal age-specific risks for trisomies at 9–14 weeks' gestation. Prenat Diagn 1994;14:543–52.

[6] Merkatz IR, Nitowsky HM, Macri JN, et al. An association between low maternal serum α-fetoprotein and fetal chromosomal abnormalities. Am J Obstet Gynecol 1984;148:886–94.

[7] Bogart MH, Pandian MR, Jones OW. Abnormal maternal serum chorionic gonadotropins levels in pregnancies with fetal chromosome abnormalities. Prenat Diagn 1987;7:623–30.

[8] Canick JA, Knight GJ, Palomaki GE, et al. Low serum trimester maternal serum unconjugated estriol in pregnancies with Down's syndrome. Br J Obstet Gynaecol 1988;95:330–3.

[9] Wald NJ, Cuckle HS, Densem JW, et al. Maternal serum screening for Down's syndrome in early pregnancy. BMJ 1988;297:883–7.

[10] Nicolaides KH, Azar G, Byrne D, et al. Fetal nuchal translucency: ultrasound screening for chromosomal defects in first trimester of pregnancy. BMJ 1992;304:867–89.

[11] Snijders RJM, Noble P, Sebire JN, et al. UK multicentre project on assessment of risk of trisomy 21 by maternal age and fetal nuchal translucency thickness at 10–14 weeks of gestation. Lancet 1998;351:343–6.

[12] Bindra R, Heath V, Liao A, et al. One-stop clinic for assessment of risk of trisomy 21 at 11–14 weeks: a prospective study of 15030 pregnancies. Ultrasound Obstet Gynecol 2002;20: 219–25.

[13] Spencer K, Souter V, Tul N, et al. A screening program for trisomy 21 at 10–14 weeks using fetal nuchal translucency, maternal serum free β-human chorionic gonadotropin and pregnancy-associated plama protein-A. Ultrasound Obstet Gynecol 1999;13:231–7.

[14] Cicero S, Curcio P, Papageorghiou A, et al. Absence of nasal bone in fetuses with trisomy 21 at 11–14 weeks of gestation: an observational study. Lancet 2001;358:1665–7.

[15] Spencer K, Salonen R, Muller F. Down's syndrome screening in multiple pregnancies using alpha-fetoprotein and free beta hCG. Prenat Diagn 1994;18:537–42.

[16] Sebire NJ, D'Ercole C, Hughes K, et al. Increased nuchal translucency thickness at 10–14 weeks of gestation as a predictor of severe twin-to-twin transfusion syndrome. Ultrasound Obstet Gynecol 1997;10:86–9.

[17] Myrianthopoulos NC. Congenital malformations: the contribution of twin studies. Birth Defects Orig Artic Ser 1978;14:151–65.

[18] Baldwin VJ. Anomalous development of twins. In: Baldwin VJ, editor. Pathology of multiple pregnancy. New York: Springer-Verlag; 1994. p. 169–97.

[19] Rodis JF, Egan JF, Craffey A, et al. Calculated risk of chromosomal abnormalities in twin gestations. Obstet Gynecol 1990;76:1037–41.

[20] Cuckle H. Down's syndrome screening in twins. J Med Screen 1998;5:3–4.

[21] Fisk NM, Bennett PR. Prenatal determination of chorionicity and zygosity. In: Ward RH, Whittle W, editors. Multiple pregnancy. London: RCOG Press; 1995. p. 56–66.

[22] Meyers C, Adam R, Dungan J, et al. Aneuploidy in twin gestations: when is maternal age advanced? Obstet Gynecol 1997;89:248–51.

[23] Pretorious D, Budorick N, Sciosia A, et al. Twin pregnancies in the second trimester in an α-fetoprotein screening program: sonographic evaluation and outcome. AJR Am J Roentgenol 1993;161:1007–13.

[24] Wood SL, St. Onge R, Connors G, et al. Evaluation of the twin peak sign in determining chorionicity in multiple pregnancy. Obstet Gynecol 1996;88:6–9.

[25] Sepulveda W, Sebire N, Hughes K, et al. The lambda sign at 10–14 weeks of gestation as a predictor of chorionicity in twin pregnancies. Ultrasound Obstet Gynecol 1996;7:421–3.

[26] Sepulveda W, Sebire N, Hughes K, et al. Evolution of the lambda or twin-chorionic peak sign in dichorionic twin pregnancies. Obstet Gynecol 1997;89:439–41.

[27] Jenkins TM, Wapner RJ. The challenge of prenatal diagnosis in twin pregnancies. Curr Opin Obstet Gynecol 2000;12:87–92.

[28] Wenstrom KD, Syrop CH, Hammitt DG, et al. Increased risk of monochorionic twinning associated with assisted reproduction. Fertil Steril 1993;60:510–4.

[29] Blickstein I, Verhoeven HC, Keith LG. Zygotic splitting after assisted reproduction. N Engl J Med 1999;340:738–9.

[30] Spencer K. Screening for trisomy 21 in twin pregnancies in the first trimester: does chorionicity impact on maternal serum free beta-hCG or PAPP-A levels. Prenat Diagn 2001;21:715–7.

[31] Wald NJ, Demsen JW. Maternal serum free beta-hCG in twin pregnancies: implications for screening for Down's screening. Prenat Diagn 1994;14:319–20.

[32] Wald NJ, George L, Smith D, et al. Serum screening for Down's syndrome between 8 and 14 weeks of pregnancy. Br J Obstet Gynaecol 1996;103:407–12.

[33] Spencer K. Screening for trisomy 21 in twin pregnancies in the first trimester using free β-hCG and PAPP-A, combined with fetal nuchal translucency thickness. Prenat Diagn 2000; 20:91–5.

[34] Wald NJ, Rish S, Hackshaw AK. Combining nuchal translucency and serum markers in prenatal screening for Down syndrome in twin pregnancies. Prenat Diagn 2003;23:588–92.

[35] Raty R, Virtanen A, Koskinen P, et al. Maternal midtrimester serum AFP and free beta-hCG in in vitro fertilization twin pregnancies. Prenat Diagn 2000;20:221–3.

[36] Pandya PP, Hilber F, Snijdrs RJM, et al. Nuchal translucency thickness, crown-rump length in twin pregnancies with chromosomally normal fetuses. J Ultrasound Med 1995;14:565–8.

[37] Sebire NJ, Snijders RJM, Hughes K, et al. Screening for trisomy 21 in twin pregnancies by maternal age and fetal nuchal translucency thickness at 10–14 weeks of gestation. Br J Obstet Gynaecol 1996;103:999–1003.

[38] Sebire NJ, Noble PL, Psarra A, et al. Fetal karyotyping in twin pregnancies: selection of technique by measurement of fetal nuchal translucency. Br J Obstet Gynaecol 1996;103:887–90.

[39] Sebire NJ, Souka A, Skentou H, et al. Early prediction of severe twin-twin transfusion syndrome. Hum Reprod 2000;15:2008–10.

[40] Matias A, Montenegro N, Areias JC. Anticipating twin-twin transfusion syndrome in mono-chorionic twin pregnancy: is there a role for nuchal translucency and ductus venosus blood flow evaluation at 11–14 weeks? Twin Res 2000;3:65–70.

[41] Barnabei V, Krantz DA, Macri JN, et al. Enhanced twin pregnancy detection within an open neural tube defect and Down syndrome screening protocol using free beta hCG and AFP. Prenat Diagn 1995;15:1131–4.

[42] Brambati B, Macri JN, Tului L, et al. First trimester aneuploidy screening: maternal serum PAPP-A and free beta-hCG. In: Grudzinskas JG, Ward RHT, editors. Screening for Down syndrome in the first trimester. London: RCOG Press; 1997. p. 135–47.

[43] Maymon R, Dreazen E, Rozinsky S, et al. The feasibility of nuchal translucency measurement in higher order multiple gestation achieved by assisted reproduction. Hum Reprod 1999;14: 2102–5.

[44] Montenegro N, Matias A, Areias JC, et al. Increased nuchal translucency: possible involvement of early cardiac failure. Ultrasound Obstet Gynecol 1997;10:265–8.

[45] Matias A, Gomes C, Flack N, et al. Screening for chromosomal defects at 11–14 weeks: the role of ductus venosus blood flow. Ultrasound Obstet Gynecol 1998;12:380–4.

[46] Matias A, Ramalho C, Montenegro N. Search for haemodynamic compromise at 11–14 weeks in monochorionic twin pregnancy: is abnormal flow in the ductus venosus predictive of twin-to-twin transfusion syndrome? J Maternal-Fetal Neonatal Medicine, in press.

[47] Spencer K, Nicolaides KH. Screening for trisomy 21 in twins using first trimester ultrasound and maternal serum biochemistry in a one stop clinic: a review of three years experience. Br J Obstet Gynaecol 2003;110:276–80.

ELSEVIER
SAUNDERS

Obstet Gynecol Clin N Am
32 (2005) 97–103

OBSTETRICS AND
GYNECOLOGY
CLINICS
OF NORTH AMERICA

Invasive Genetic Diagnosis in
Multiple Pregnancies

Zvi Appelman, MD[a,b,*], Boris Furman, MD[a]

[a]*Department of Obstetrics and Gynecology, Kaplan Medical Center, Rehovot 76100, Israel*
[b]*Institute of Clinical Genetics, Kaplan Medical Center, Rehovot, Israel*

The incidence of multifetal pregnancies has increased exponentially during the past two decades, mostly because of assisted reproductive technologies [1]. Typically, pregnant women who seek assisted reproductive technologies are often older, which is when the age-related risk of aneuploidy is often significant. The likelihood of at least one twin having a chromosomal abnormality is five to three times higher than in singleton pregnancies [2]. The decision to undergo prenatal diagnosis in multiple gestations is complex, and one must consider not only the risk of aneuploidy but also the procedure-related hazards. Abnormal results sometimes require selective termination of an affected sibling, a procedure that entails moral, ethical, and medical implications.

Determining chorionicity

Determination of chorionicity is crucial in assessing the perinatal risk and the risk of aneuploidy [3]. It also helps in the perinatal risk assessment [4]. The age-related risk of monozygotic twins to be simultaneously abnormal is the same as for singletons. For dizygotic twins, the probability of both twins being chromosomally abnormal is the product of their separate probabilities, this risk is relatively small. For example, the age-related risk of a 40-year-old woman having a child with Down syndrome is 1:100 for singletons; however, for dizygotic twins the probability for both children to have Down syndrome is

* Corresponding author. Department of Obstetrics and Gynecology, Kaplan Medical Center, Rehovot 76100, Israel.
E-mail address: edith_ap@yahoo.com (Z. Appelman).

0889-8545/05/$ – see front matter © 2005 Elsevier Inc. All rights reserved.
doi:10.1016/j.ogc.2004.10.003

obgyn.theclinics.com

1:100 × 1:100 = 1:10,000. First trimester ultrasound is currently accepted as the most accurate determination for chorionicity. Identification of twin-peak sign in dichorionic twins provides 100% accuracy in the first trimester [5]. In the first trimester, 100% accuracy is noted by counting the dividing membrane layers [6], and dichorionic twins have a thick chorionic inter-twin septum. In the mid-trimester, after fusion between the chorion and amnion, the accuracy in determining chorionicity is approximately 90% [7]. Other techniques for determining chorionicity (eg, septal thickness measurement and inter-twin membranes layer counting) are less popular and seem to depend on operator skills and the transducer that is used [8,9].

Invasive diagnostic procedures

When considering an invasive diagnostic procedure, adverse effects, such as procedure-related fetal loss, are weighed against the probability of an abnormal result. The accuracy of the procedure is also important. Conventional approaches include second-trimester amniocentesis or first-trimester chorionic villus sampling (CVS). The gestational age at which the diagnosis is made should be considered because most patients favor an early diagnosis. In multiple pregnancies, early diagnosis also enables the possibility of early decision making concerning selective termination or pregnancy termination.

The amniocentesis approach initially was described by Elias et al [10]. The procedure is routinely performed between 16 and 20 weeks' gestation. An ultrasound is performed for appropriate fetal measurements, number and location of each placenta, and location and characteristics of the dividing membrane. A 22-gauge needle is inserted under continuous ultrasound guidance into one sac, fluid is retrieved, 1 to 2 mL of inert dye (indigo carmine) is injected, and the needle is removed. In the same fashion, a second needle is inserted into the second twin sac under ultrasound guidance, and clear, dye-free fluid is retrieved.

With improvement of ultrasound technology and diagnostic performance skills, another technique for amniocentesis sampling has been proposed without the use of dye [11,12]. In this technique, initial ultrasound examination visualizes both sacs and the dividing membrane in the same plane. A needle is inserted into the first sac, fluid is retrieved, and the needle is pushed through the dividing membrane into the second sac under direct visualization. Using this technique, misdiagnosis can occur because of the possibility of sampling of the same sac twice or causing cell contamination.

Monochorionic pregnancy sampling provides an additional challenge. Both fetuses originate from the same zygote in the monochorionic-monozygotic gestation, and each fetus karyotype should be exactly alike. Therefore, sampling of both sacs is not recommended. There are rare cases in which monochorionic gestations may have discordant chromosomal results, the main reason being that there is no reliable method to confirm definitely that the pregnancy is monochorionic. Postzygotic non-disjunction can lead to monozygotic gestation with discordant karyotype. Because of the rarity of these events, most physicians do not recommend sampling both sacs when ultrasound findings are characteristic for monochorionic twins.

Loss rates after amniocentesis in multiple gestations

No randomized control trials have been conducted regarding the safety of amniocentesis in multiple gestations. Fig. 1 shows the pregnancy loss rates before 20 and 28 weeks' gestation in various studies [12–20]. Pregnancy loss rates in these studies ranged from 0 to 6% up to 20 weeks and from 0 to 8% up to 28 weeks. Overall, the mean pregnancy loss up to 20 weeks' gestation is 1.9% and up to 28 weeks it is 3.5%. The risk of pregnancy loss before 28 weeks' gestation in unsampled twins after a normal second-trimester ultrasound is 4.5% to 7.2% [21]. In their case-control study, Ghidini et al [18] reported similar pregnancy loss rates between twins and their gestational age-matched unsampled controls—3% versus 2.8%, respectively. The rate of procedure-related pregnancy loss after amniocentesis in twin pregnancies is not different from that of singletons and is empirically estimated to be approximately 1%. In a retrospective study, that involved 476 women with bichorionic twins who underwent amniocentesis and 477 untested twins, Yukobowich et al [22] found statistically significant differences between pregnancy loss rates 4 weeks after the amniocentesis—2.7% versus 0.6% ($P = 0.01$), respectively. In recent study,

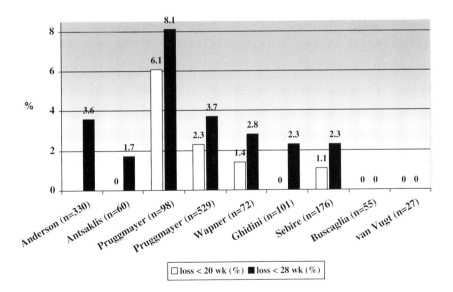

Fig. 1. Pregnancy loss rates after amniocentesis in twins. (*Data from* Refs. [12–20].)

Toth-Pal et al [23] also compared the spontaneous pregnancy losses between 175 women with twins after amniocentesis and 300 twin pairs as controls. They found that spontaneous losses in multiple pregnancies between weeks 18 and 24 were 2.39%, whereas if amniocentesis was performed, the loss rate before the week 24 was 3.87%. Despite a nonsignificant statistical difference, they concluded that genetic amniocentesis in multiple pregnancies slightly increases the fetal loss rate until 24 weeks' gestation. Patients who undergo twin amniocentesis should be informed that there is a greater risk of pregnancy loss than in singleton pregnancies, although most cases are not related to the procedure.

Chorionic villus sampling in twins

CVS has become a safe and efficacious alternative to amniocentesis for the identification of genetic abnormalities. The standard of care is to perform CVS after 10 weeks' gestation to avoid limb reduction defects. A detailed ultrasound examination should be undertaken to determine fetal age, chorionicity, placental location, and the presence of major malformation. Performance of CVS in multiple pregnancies demands an accurate assessment of the site of placental implantation for each fetus and zygosity verification. Transcervical and transabdominal approaches are used for carrying out this procedure [24]. Some pitfalls exist when performing CVS. There is no apparent way to secure sampling of each frondosum site; therefore, the same fetus can be sampled twice involuntarily. Inter-twin villi contamination and sampling errors occur in approximately 4% of samples [25]. One study compared the diagnostic accuracy of amniocentesis and CVS in twins and triplets [26]. Second-trimester amniocentesis was performed in 297 women and CVS in 163. Successful sampling with two-pass approach was achieved in 99.3% versus 99.7%, respectively. Uncertain results were present in seven CVS cases (five of which involved placental mosaicism). No uncertain results were found in the group that underwent amniocentesis. In 15 triplet sets, 4 were sampled by CVS and 11 underwent amniocentesis; however, 1 from each group required further amniocentesis because of abnormal results. The authors concluded that clinical questions caused by fetal cell contamination and confined placental mosaicism can be kept to a minimum with CVS and do not lead to mistakes of critical importance.

Loss rates after chorionic villus sampling in multiple gestations

First-trimester CVS in multiple gestation seems to have pregnancy loss rates comparable to that of amniocentesis. Fig. 2 represents pregnancy loss rates after CVS in twins. According to the included studies [17,24,25,27], the rate of

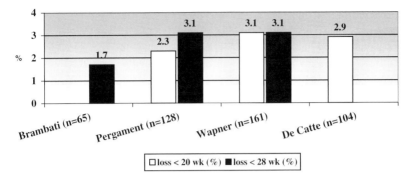

Fig. 2. Pregnancy loss rates after CVS in twins. (*Data from* Refs. [17,24,25,27].)

pregnancy loss up to 20 weeks after CVS is 2.3% to 3.1%, whereas up to 28 weeks the rate is 1.7% to 3.1%. Overall, in total 458 twin pairs, the pregnancy loss rates before 20 and 28 weeks' gestation were alike (2.8%). Wapner et al [17] compared the procedure-related loss rates between first-trimester CVS and second-trimester amniocentesis. The fetal loss rate after the procedure until 28 weeks' gestation was 2.9% after amniocentesis and 3.2% after CVS. Altogether the total fetal loss (corrected for the abnormal fetuses) was found to be 9.3% after amniocentesis and only 4.9% after CVS. Researchers concluded that CVS is at least as safe and reliable as amniocentesis for prenatal diagnosis of twin pregnancies.

Fig. 3 shows reported outcomes of CVS in twin pregnancies according to pregnancy losses before 22 weeks' gestation and total fetal loss. Of 614 twin pregnancies, the mean rate of pregnancy losses before 22 weeks' gestation was 3.1%, and mean total pregnancy loss was 4.6% [28].

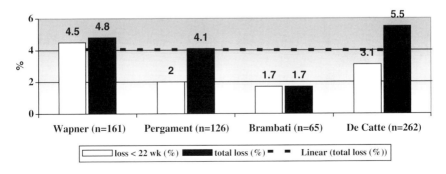

Fig. 3. Outcome of CVS in twins. (*Data from* Refs. [17,24,25,28].)

Summary

Invasive testing using CVS or amniocentesis can be performed safely in multiple gestations. Preprocedural counseling must apply to the particular aspects for multiple gestations. Overall, CVS for multiple pregnancies has many advantages. In twins, it seems that CVS and amniocentesis carry a similar fetal loss rate. CVS also leads to early and accurate results. Selective reduction, when indicated, can be performed in the first trimester rather than in the second trimester, which reduces fetal losses. Only experienced centers should perform these procedures because of technical skills needed. In conclusion, prenatal diagnosis in multifetal pregnancy by CVS is safe, accurate, and effective. It seems that CVS should be the procedure of choice in most cases.

References

[1] Evans MI, Littmann L, St Louis L, et al. Evolving patterns of iatrogenic multifetal pregnancy generation: implications for aggressiveness of infertility treatments. Am J Obstet Gynecol 1995; 172:1750–3.

[2] Rodis JF, Egan JF, Craffey A, et al. Calculated risk of chromosomal abnormalities in twin gestations. Obstet Gynecol 1990;76:1037–41.

[3] Fisk MN, Bryan E. Routine prenatal determination of chorionicity in multiple gestation: a plea to the obstetrician. Br J Obstet Gynaecol 1993;100:975–7.

[4] Sebire NJ, Snijders RJM, Hughes K, et al. The hidden mortality of monochorionic twin pregnancies. Br J Obstet Gynaecol 1997;104:1203–7.

[5] Sepulveda W, Sebine NJ, Hughes K, et al. Evolution of the lambda or twin-chorionic peak sign in dichorionic twin pregnancies. Obstet Gynecol 1997;89:439–41.

[6] Monteagudo A, Timor-Tritsch IE, Sharma S. Early and simple determination of chorionic and amniotic type in multifetal gestations in the first fourteen weeks by high-frequency transvaginal ultrasonography. Am J Obstet Gynecol 1994;170:824–9.

[7] Wood SL, St Orange R, Connors G, et al. Evaluation of the twin peak or lambda sign in determining chorionicity in multiple pregnancy. Obstet Gynecol 1996;88:6–9.

[8] Stagiannis KD, Sepulveda W, Southwell D, et al. Ultrasonographic measurements of the dividing membrane in twin pregnancy during the second and third trimesters: a reproducibility study. Am J Obstet Gynecol 1995;173:1546–50.

[9] Vayssiere CF, Heim N, Camus EP, et al. Determination of chorionicity in twin gestations by high-frequency abdominal ultrasonography: counting the layers of the dividing membrane. Am J Obstet Gynecol 1996;175:1529–33.

[10] Elias S, Gerbie A, Simpson JL, et al. Genetic amniocentesis in twin gestations. Am J Obstet Gynecol 1980;138:169–74.

[11] Jeanty P, Shah D, Roussis P. Single-needle insertion in twin amniocentesis. J Ultrasound Med 1990;9:511–7.

[12] Sebire MJ, Noble PL, Odibo A, et al. Single uterine entry for genetic amniocentesis in twin pregnancies. Lancet 1996;47:26–31.

[13] Anderson RL, Goldenberg JD, Golbus MS. Prenatal diagnosis in multiple gestation: 20 years' experience with amniocentesis. Prenat Diagn 1991;11:263–70.

[14] Antsaklis A, Gougoulakis A, Mesogitis S, et al. Invasive techniques for fetal diagnosis in multiple pregnancy. Int J Gynaecol Obstet 1991;34:309–14.

[15] Pruggmayer M, Baumann P, Schutte H, et al. Incidence of abortion after genetic amniocentesis in twin pregnancies. Prenat Diagn 1991;11:637–40.

[16] Pruggmayer MRK, Jahoda MGJ, Van der Pol JG, et al. Genetic amniocentesis in twin pregnancies: results of a multicenter study of 529 cases. Ultrasound Obstet Gynecol 1992;2:6–10.

[17] Wapner RJ, Jonhson A, Davis G. Prenatal diagnosis in twin gestation: a comparison between second trimester amniocentesis and first trimester chorionic villus sampling. Obstet Gynecol 1993;82:49–56.

[18] Ghidini A, Lynch L, Hicks C, et al. The risk of second-trimester amniocentesis in twin gestations: a case-control study. Am J Obstet Gynecol 1993;169:1013–6.

[19] Buscaglia M, Chisoni L, Bellotti M, et al. Genetic amniocentesis in biamniotic twin pregnancies by a single transabdominal insertion of the needle. Prenat Diagn 1995;15:17–9.

[20] Van Vugt M, Nieuwint A, van Geijn HP. Single-needle insertion: an alternative technique for early second-trimester genetic twin amniocentesis. Fetal Diagn Ther 1995;10:178–81.

[21] Pretorious D, Budorick N, Sciossia A, et al. Twin pregnancies in the second trimester in an α-fetoprotein screening program: sonographic evaluation and outcome. AJR Am J Roentgenol 1993;161:1007–13.

[22] Yukobowich E, Anteby EY, Cohen SM, et al. Risk of fetal loss in twin pregnancies undergoing second trimester amniocentesis. Obstet Gynecol 2001;98:231–4.

[23] Toth-Pal E, Papp C, Beke A, et al. Genetic amniocentesis in multiple pregnancies. Fetal Diagn Ther 2004;19:138–44.

[24] Brambati B, Tului L, Lanzana A, et al. First trimester genetic diagnosis in multiple pregnancies: principals and potential pitfalls. Prenat Diagn 1991;11:767–74.

[25] Pergament E, Schulman J, Copeland K, et al. The risk of and efficacy of chorionic villus sampling in multiple gestation. Prenat Diagn 1992;12:377–84.

[26] Van den Berg C, Braat APG, Van Opstal D, et al. Amniocentesis or chorionic villus sampling in multiple gestations? Experience with 500 cases. Prenat Diagn 1999;19:234–44.

[27] De Catte L, Liebaers I, Foulon W, et al. First trimester chorionic villus sampling in twin gestations. Am J Perinatol 1996;13:413–7.

[28] De Catte L, Liebaers I, Foulon W. Outcome of twin gestations after first trimester chorionic villus sampling. Obstet Gynecol 2000;95:714–20.

ELSEVIER
SAUNDERS

Obstet Gynecol Clin N Am
32 (2005) 105–126

OBSTETRICS AND
GYNECOLOGY
CLINICS
OF NORTH AMERICA

Invasive Antenatal Interventions in Complicated Multiple Pregnancies

Liesbeth Lewi, MD[a],*, Jacques Jani, MD[b], Jan Deprest, MD, PhD[a]

[a]*Department of Obstetrics and Gynecology, University Hospital Gasthuisberg, Herestraat 49, B-3000 Leuven, Belgium*
[b]*Centre for Surgical Technologies, Minderbroederstraat 17, B-3000 Leuven, Belgium*

Twins have a more complicated in utero stay than singletons. Management also is complicated by the fact that more than one fetus must be taken into account and varies according to chorionicity. Approximately 30% of twins are monozygotic and 70% are dizygotic. Monozygotic twins result from the fertilization of a single egg followed by early division into two cell masses, which further develop separately. In 30%, cleavage occurs before the third day after fertilization, which results in dichorionic diamniotic twins, whereas in 70%, splitting takes place after the third day, which results in monochorionic twins in its different manifestations. Dizygotic twins result from the fertilization of two different eggs. By definition, dizygotic twins are dichorionic and diamniotic (Fig. 1). Correct determination of chorionicity is paramount to correct management of multiple pregnancies and is highly accurate when performed in the first trimester (Fig. 2) [1].

Monochorionic multiples run the highest risk of complications, and the well-being of one fetus crucially depends on that of the other(s) because of the almost ever-present vascular anastomoses in the common placenta (Fig. 3) [2]. These vascular anastomoses can cause significant blood volume shifts between the fetuses, which lead to complications such as twin-to-twin transfusion syndrome (TTTS), twin reversed arterial perfusion (TRAP), and acute exsanguination of the

Drs. Lewi and Jani received a grant from the European Commission in its fifth Framework Programme (#QLG1-CT-2002-01632 EuroTwin2Twin).

* Corresponding author.
E-mail address: Liesbeth.Lewi@uz.kuleuven.ac.be (L. Lewi).

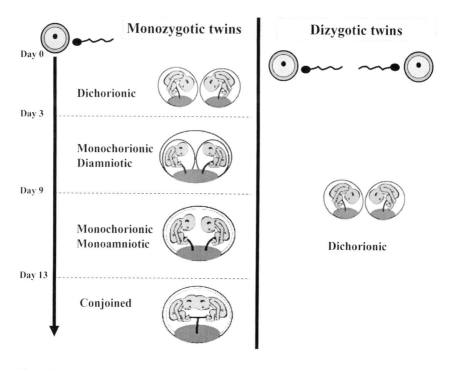

Fig. 1. Zygosity and chorionicity in twin pregnancies. Arrow depicts number of days after fertilization.

survivor in the fetoplacental unit at the time of demise of its co-twin. Sono-endoscopic surgery on the placenta and the umbilical cord plays an important role in the treatment of certain complicated monochorionic multiple pregnancies and has acquired an established place in modern fetal medicine [3]. TTTS affects approximately 10% to 15% of monochorionic twins, and fetoscopic laser treatment of the vascular anastomoses is currently the best treatment available [4]. For selective feticide in monochorionic multiple pregnancies, the conventional method of potassium chloride injection into the target fetus' circulation is unsuitable because the toxic drug may embolize to the healthy fetus(es). Patent anastomoses can trigger acute exsanguination of the surviving fetus into the demised fetus' circulation [5]. Minimally invasive techniques have been developed to separate and occlude the sacrificed fetus' circulation completely and permanently [6].

Fetoscopic laser treatment for twin-to-twin transfusion syndrome

In nearly all monochorionic multiple pregnancies, interfetal transfusion is a constant but usually balanced phenomenon. In approximately 10% to 15%, however, a chronic imbalance in net flow develops, which results in TTTS. The donor twin becomes hypovolemic, and develops oliguria and oligohydramnios,

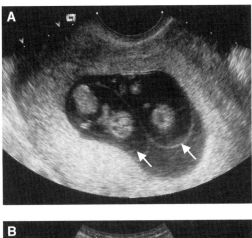

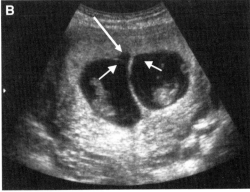

Fig. 2. Chorionicity determination on the first trimester ultrasound scan. (*A*) Monochorionic diamniotic twins. Only two thin amniotic membranes (*arrows*) separate the two fetuses. (*B*) Dichorionic diamniotic twins. The fetuses are separated by three layers (amnion, chorion-chorion, amnion).

also known as the "stuck twin" sequence. Hypervolemia, polyuria, and polyhydramnios evolve in the recipient twin, who can develop circulatory overload and hydrops. TTTS typically occurs between 15 and 26 weeks' gestation and is a sonographic diagnosis based on the following criteria:

- Polyhydramnios in the sac of the recipient twin (defined as deepest vertical pocket of $\geq$ 8cm before 20 weeks and $\geq$ 10 cm between 20 and 26 weeks) with signs of polyuria (distended bladder)
- Oligohydramnios in the donor's sac (deepest vertical pocket $\leq$ 2cm) with signs of oliguria (small or empty bladder) (Fig. 4)

Discordant growth may be present but is not a prerequisite for the diagnosis. The pathophysiology of TTTS is usually explained on an angioarchitectural basis. Placental anastomoses can be arterio-arterial, arteriovenous (AV), and veno-venous or a combination of these types [7]. Arterio-arterial and veno-venous

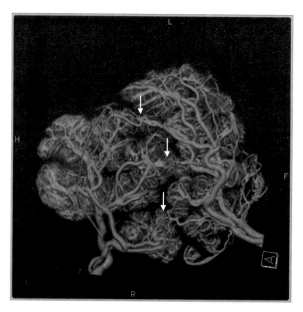

Fig. 3. Three-dimensional reconstruction of a CT angiogram of a monochorionic placenta at term shows an equal distribution of the placental mass and a large arterio-arterial and veno-venous superficial anastomosis (*arrows*). (In collaboration with M. Cannie, Department of Radiology, Leuven, Belgium.)

anastomoses are typically superficial, bi-directional anastomoses on the surface of the chorionic plate that form direct communications between the arteries and veins of the two fetal circulations. AV anastomoses occur at the capillary level, deep within a shared cotyledon, and receive arterial supply from one twin and provide venous drainage to the other twin. The supplying artery and draining vein

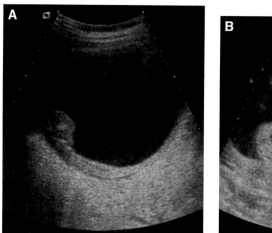
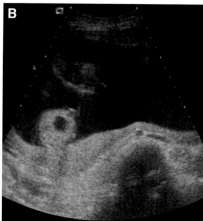

Fig. 4. Ultrasound image of TTTS. (*A*) The donor is stuck to the uterine wall without bladder filling. (*B*) Hydramnios is present in the sac of the recipient, who has a distended bladder.

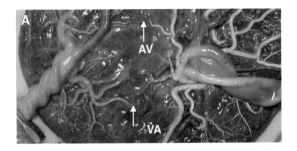

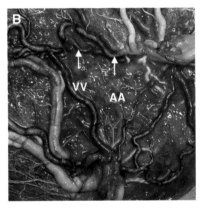

Fig. 5. Macroscopic image after dye injection of a monochorionic placenta. (*A*) An AV and oppositely directed VA anastomosis. (*B*) A superficial AA and VV anastomosis.

of the AV anastomosis can be visualized on the placental surface, where they pierce the chorionic plate at close proximity to each other to supply the shared cotyledon, which also may receive other vessels (Fig. 5). AV anastomoses allow flow in one direction only and can create an imbalance in the interfetal transfusion that leads to TTTS unless balanced by an oppositely directed transfusion through other (superficial or deep) anastomoses.

Untreated, severe, mid-gestational TTTS has a mortality rate of nearly 100%. Polyhydramnios may lead to spontaneous abortion, rupture of the membranes, or extreme preterm delivery, and fetal death may result from cardiac failure in the recipient or poor perfusion in the donor. There are also substantial risks of cerebral and cardiac sequelae in survivors because of the chronic hemodynamic imbalance. Initially, only serial amnioreduction was available as a treatment option to reduce the polyhydramnios and intrauterine pressure, thus alleviating symptoms and prolonging pregnancy and having some beneficial effects on fetoplacental perfusion. Repeated amnioreduction is a simple and widely available technique, but it does not address the vascular basis of TTTS. The anastomoses remain patent, and in the event of a single intrauterine fetal death (IUFD), the surviving twin is at high risk of IUFD, anemia, and neurologic damage. Vascular anastomoses can be visualized on the chorionic surface during fetoscopy, and their coagulation could be a causative treatment. A recent randomized trial set up by members of the Eurofoetus research consortium compared serial amnioreduction versus laser coagulation for severe TTTS before 26 weeks' gestation. The research showed that laser had significantly better outcome in terms of survival of at least one twin (76% versus 51%), gestational age at delivery (33.3 weeks' versus 29 weeks' gestation), and neurologic damage (6% versus 14%) [4]. Laser therefore appears to be a better first-line treatment than amnioreduction.

Technique of laser coagulation

Hardware

Minimal investments into good-quality, video-endoscopic hardware are a prerequisite, including a high-quality light fountain, video camera and monitor, and purpose-designed fetoscopes. Appropriate energy sources are needed to coagulate the vessels of interest. For laser, an Nd:YAG (minimal power requirements 60–100 W) or diode laser (minimal power requirements 30–60 W) with fibers of 400 to 600 μm suffice; the electrosurgical generator is standard equipment.

Fetoscopic endoscopes differ from their hysteroscopic or laparoscopic counterparts but are delivered by the same suppliers. Currently, the experience gathered with any type of fetoscope is limited and no evidence shows that one particular brand of endoscope performs better than another. Intuitively, one strives for a combination of minimal diameter, appropriate length, and maximal resolution. Personal preference, local factors such as after sales-service, and compatibility with other operation room equipment influence the choice of the manufacturer. In Europe, considerable investments have been made by the European Commission in its "Biomed 2 Programme" for instrument development by a partner of the Eurofoetus research consortium (Karl Storz Endoskope) [8]. Thanks to this project, a range of 20- to 30-cm fetoscopes with diameters of 1 to 2.3 mm are currently available (Fig. 6). Most of the scopes are semi-flexible 0° fiber-optic scopes that can be curved (eg, to direct the scope toward an anteriorly located placenta) [9]. More typical rod lens telescopes also have been fabricated, with angles of inclination up to 30° and an associated deflecting mechanism for the laser fiber. Steerable fiber scopes have been used for an anterior placenta [10,11]; however, image quality is not optimal because of poor light transmission (unpublished observations). All scopes are used within a sheath that houses the endoscope and any additional instruments, such as a laser fiber. Fibers are usually inserted through an additional working channel to keep the fiber in a stable position. Luer lock connections allow irrigation or drainage of fluid.

To gain entry, the sheath can be introduced either directly or through a cannula. For direct introduction, the sheath is loaded with its accompanying trocar. The sheath is inserted into the amniotic cavity under ultrasound guidance. Once inside, the trocar is removed and is replaced by the fetoscope. During the procedure, the sheath can be moved back and forth but cannot be withdrawn without losing access to the amniotic cavity. The use of formal cannulae obviates this problem because the port remains in place during the entire procedure and

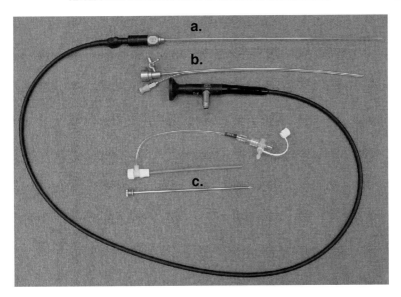

Fig. 6. Example of fetoscopic instruments as used for laser coagulation of the vascular anastomoses in TTTS. (*a*) Straightforward telescope: diameter 2 mm, length 30 cm, with remote eyepiece (Karl Storz, Tuttlingen, Germany). (*b*) Fetoscopic sheath with channel for laser fibers up to 600 μm with one stopcock and one Luer-lock adaptor (Karl Storz). (*c*) Cannula (Cook Surgical, Bloomington, IN) with purposely developed trocar (Karl Storz).

instruments and scopes can be introduced numerous times. We use thin-walled cannulae that are semi-flexible to accommodate curved instruments and come in various sizes with purpose-developed fitting trocars. Currently no data are available to support either the direct or cannula access method to the amniotic cavity. Further technical details on endoscopes and ancillary equipment are available in more recent handbooks on fetal therapy [12–14].

Procedure

In our institution, preoperatively all patients receive 2 g cefazolin intravenously and 20 mg slow-release nifedipin orally. Laser coagulation is performed by percutaneous approach (Fig. 7) through a 3-mm incision under local or locoregional anesthesia and under strict aseptic conditions. The position of the fetuses, umbilical cord insertions, and placenta is mapped by ultrasound scan. A skin incision is made to accommodate the sheath, and under ultrasound guidance the cannula or fetoscopic sheath is inserted into the hydramniotic sac (Fig. 8). At all times, the placenta, fetal parts, maternal vessels, and bowel are avoided.

In twin-to-twin transfusion, fetoscopic detection of the anastomoses is improved by the presence of polyhydramnios, which flattens the placenta. Occasionally, however, vision may be hampered by blood or debris. In these instances, amnio-exchange with warmed Hartmann's solution heated by a blood warmer or a special amnio-irrigator can improve visibility [15]. Three fixed landmarks are available to identify any anastomosing vessels: (1) the intertwin membrane,

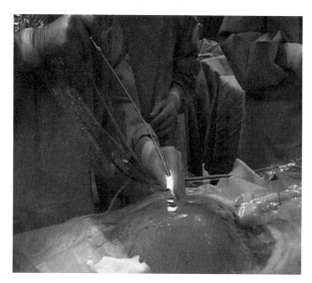

Fig. 7. Image of the operative set-up and percutaneous access used for fetoscopic interventions.

(2) the recipient's cord insertion, and (3) the donor's cord insertion. The intertwin septum and its placental insertion are easily identified as a white line (Fig. 9). From there, blood vessels that leave the donor usually cross under the septum in the direction of the recipient. These blood vessels are followed to identify any anastomosing vessels. The vascular equator usually does not coincide with the intertwin septum and cannot be predicted by simple determination of the cord insertions. Alternatively, vessels also can be followed starting from the recipient's or donor's cord insertion. The purpose of the procedure is to visualize the entire

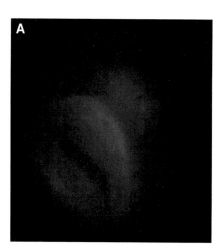
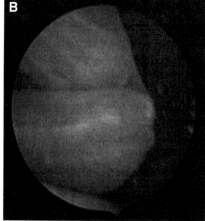

Fig. 8. (*A*) Fetoscopic image of the face of the recipient, who moves freely in the hydramniotic sac. (*B*) Fetoscopic image of the feet of the donor, who is stuck behind the intertwin septum.

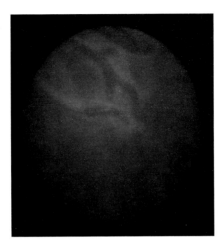

Fig. 9. Fetoscopic image of the intertwin septum inserting on the chorionic surface with the donor's vessels crossing underneath.

vascular equator and coagulate all anastomoses. A "hyperselective" approach (ie, coagulating only the causative AV anastomosis), as discussed by Feldstein et al [16], is not used in the European centers that practice laser coagulation. Any residual anastomoses put the remaining fetuses at risk of hypovolemic events in case of single IUFD and even may lead to persistence or reversal of transfusion. Arteries are distinguishable from veins because they have a darker color caused by the deoxygenated blood. Arteries usually cross over the veins.

Occasionally, it may be impossible to determine whether vessels anastomose because of the position of the intertwin septum, placenta, fetus, or other physical limitations. In these instances, the vessels also are coagulated. With an anterior placenta, the amniotic sac and the vessels on the placenta may be more difficult to access. Instruments for anterior placentas have been developed, but it is unclear whether they improve performance. So far, similar outcomes have been reported for anteriorly and posteriorly located placentas.

Coagulation is performed at a distance of approximately 1 cm and ideally at a 90° angle using a non-touch technique (Fig. 10). Sections of approximately 1 cm are coagulated with shots of approximately 3 to 4 seconds, according to tissue response. Laser energy is adapted to the source used, the diameter of the vessels, and the tissue response. Typically an Nd:YAG laser is set at 50 to 70 W and a diode laser at 30 to 40 W. Large vessels can be coagulated from various angles to obtain progressive narrowing and eventual coagulation. The use of excessive laser power levels should be avoided because it may cause vessel perforation and fetal hemorrhage. Once all vessels are coagulated, the vascular equator is followed to ascertain that all anastomoses have been coagulated fully and that flow has not resumed.

The procedure is completed by amnioreduction until normal amniotic fluid pockets are seen on ultrasound scan. The cannula or sheath is removed under

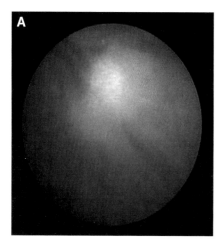
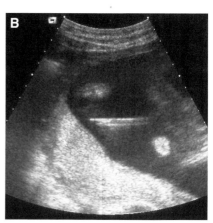

Fig. 10. (*A*) Fetoscopic image of a coagulated AV anastosomosis. (*B*) Ultrasound image during laser coagulation demonstrating the non-touch technique with the laser fiber at 1 cm distance from the chorionic plate.

ultrasound guidance to detect any significant bleeding from the uterine wall. Postoperatively, the patient remains as an inpatient for 48 hours. Blood pressure, pulse, temperature, and fluid balance are monitored. Ultrasound scanning is repeated the first and second day to document fetal viability, Doppler, amniotic fluid volume, and bladder filling. Cefazolin is repeated every 8 hours for 24 hours, and the patient continues to take oral nifedepin every 12 hours for 48 hours.

Risks and outcome of the procedure

In contrast to amnioreduction, in which IUFD of one or both fetuses often occurs remotely from the procedure, most IUFD procedures with laser are diagnosed within 48 hours. In our experience of the first 100 cases, this happens in 18% and affects the donor as often as the recipient. The cause of these deaths remains largely unexplained, although it is generally assumed that too little placental mass may remain after laser for both fetuses to survive [17]. Preliminary data suggest that preoperative MRI accurately predicts placental distribution in TTTS and that postoperative IUFD is not restricted to the fetus with the smallest placental mass [18]. Further research is needed regarding the exact cause of these losses. The surviving twin seems far less likely to be anemic after laser [19] or to sustain neurologic sequelae [20,21] compared with survivors after amnioreduction in which the anastomoses remain patent.

Another important fetal risk is preterm delivery. In the Eurofoetus randomized, controlled trial, median gestational age at delivery was higher in the laser than in the amnioreduction group (33.3 weeks' versus 29 weeks' gestation), with 42% and 69% women, respectively, delivering before 32 weeks. Preterm prelabor rupture of the membranes (PPROM) remains the most important complication of invasive antenatal procedures and accounts for a high morbidity and mortality if the membranes rupture before viability. In our own initial experience (n = 100), PPROM within 5 weeks of the procedure occurred in 16%. The overall incidence of PPROM before 37 weeks was 45% with median gestational age at delivery of 30 weeks in cases with PPROM compared with 35 weeks in causes without PPROM. The intra-amniotic injection of platelets and clotting factors may be a successful technique to treat cases of early postoperative PPROM [22,23]. Other rare fetal complications include congenital skin loss, gangrenous limb lesions, microphthalmia, and intestinal atresia [24,25]. These anomalies have been de-scribed in TTTS not treated by laser [26] and also can originate from the disease process itself.

The neurologic infant outcome in laser for TTTS may be determined by the severity of the disease, the gestational age at delivery, and the procedure. In the Eurofoetus randomized, controlled trial, infants in the amnioreduction group had higher incidences of cystic periventricular leukomalacia (laser 6% versus amnio-drainage 14%), particularly the recipients. Currently, the children are being fol-lowed until 2 years of age, and results are eagerly awaited. A recent long-term, follow-up study of children who survived an uncontrolled series managed by laser (age between 14 and 44 months of age) observed major neurologic prob-lems in 11% of survivors [27].

Maternal safety remains a priority, and serious maternal complications should be noted carefully in a registry, such as the one set up by Eurofoetus [3]. Tran-sient maternal mirror or Ballantyne syndrome with pulmonary edema, placental abruption, chorioamnionitis, and bleeding that requires transfusion were reported but have not led to maternal death. In the Eurofoetus randomized, controlled trial, there was no severe maternal morbidity (no woman required intensive care unit admission or blood transfusion), although three placental abruptions occurred at the end of the amnioreduction (two in the amnioreduction and one in the laser group). The women required immediate delivery. Infection is another potential problem. Hecher et al [28] demonstrated a learning curve and argued against scattering the experience over too many centers. In our study on fertility and pregnancy outcome in a consecutive series of 100 patients, fetoscopic inter-ventions did not seem to influence future fertility and pregnancy outcome [29].

Selective feticide in multiple pregnancies

The indications, technique, and outcome of selective feticide in complicated multiple pregnancies crucially depend on an exact chorionicity determination in the first trimester. In monochorionic multiple pregnancies, selective feticide may be contemplated for several indications: (1) a severe discordant structural or chromosomal anomaly, (2) severe discordant growth with high risk of IUFD, (3) TRAP, and (4) severe TTTS with associated discordant anomaly or rare cases in which inspection of the chorionic plate was precluded by the position of the fetus and placenta. In contrast, in dichorionic twins, selective feticide is restricted to the management of discordant structural or chromosomal anomalies.

Structural anomalies are more common in twins. Unfortunately, most studies have not related their incidence to zygosity or chorionicity. It seems that in dizygotic twins, the rate per fetus is the same as in singletons, whereas in monozygotic twins the rate is two to three times higher [30]. Even in monochorionic twins, in more than 80% of cases only one fetus is affected [31]. The exact mechanism of this increased prevalence remains unknown.

In dizygotic twins, the age-related risk of chromosomal abnormalities for one twin is independent of the risk for the other and should be the same as in singletons. The risk of at least one fetus having Down syndrome theoretically should be double that in singletons. In contrast, all monochorionic twins are monozygotic, and the risk for chromosomal abnormalities should be the same as for singletons. In most cases, both fetuses are equally affected. Discordance in monochorionic twins for nearly all common human aneuploidies (trisomy 13 [32], trisomy 21 [33], monosomy 45,X [33]) has been reported. Most cases involve one twin with Turner syndrome and the other with either a female or male phenotype, but usually it is a mosaic karyotype. This rare phenomenon is called heterokaryotypic monozygotism and is related to postzygotic mitotic events (nondisjunction or anaphase lag) or prezygotic meiotic errors. Our series of selective feticide includes five such cases of discordant chromosomes in monochorionic twins (46, XY/47,XY, + 21; 46,XX/47,XX, + 13; 46,XY/45,X; two cases of 46,XX/45,X) [34]. Heterokaryotypic monochorionic twins can be diagnosed prenatally only if an amniocentesis is performed on both amniotic sacs, which is recommended in the event of discordant anomalies in monochorionic twins [34].

There are essentially three management options for discordant structural and chromosomal anomalies: conservative management, selective feticide, or termination of the whole pregnancy. For anomalies that are nonlethal but may result in serious handicap, parents must decide whether the burden of a handicapped child is enough to risk the loss of the healthy twin from feticide-related complications. In dichorionic twins and for lethal anomalies, it may be best to avoid such risk and conservative management is preferable, unless the condition threatens the well-being of the healthy twin. Such a dilemma is illustrated by twins discordant for anencephaly, which is always lethal but because of associated polyhydramnios places the healthy co-twin at risk of severe preterm delivery. Whereas in dichorionic twins expectant management may be preferable for anomalies with a high risk of in utero demise, in monochorionic twins this specifically warrants selective feticide. In dichorionic twins, single IUFD is associated with perinatal death or handicap of the surviving twin in 5% to 10% and is largely caused by extreme preterm delivery. In contrast, single IUFD in monochorionic twins has a co-twin IUFD rate of 10% to 25%. There are also antenatal cerebral lesions in 25% to 45% of surviving twins because of acute exsanguination in the fetoplacental unit of the dead twin and the effects of extreme preterm delivery [35,36].

Severe early discordant growth in monochorionic twins at high risk of IUFD of the growth-retarded twin also may constitute an indication for selective feticide to protect the surviving twin better against the adverse effects of spontaneous demise of its co-twin. Two recent series highlighted the risk of IUFD and cerebral damage in severe discordant growth [37,38]. In one series (n = 13), abnormal neurodevelopment was observed in 42% of children and cerebral palsy rates were 19% [37]. There were four instances of IUFD, three children survived, and all had cerebral palsy. The other series (n = 42) showed an IUFD rate of 10% with 12% parenchymal brain damage in surviving infants [38]. These data clearly demonstrate that monochorionic twins with discordant growth are at especially high risk of adverse outcome.

An extreme manifestation of TTTS is TRAP, which complicates approximately 1% of monochorionic twin pregnancies. In TRAP, blood flows from an umbilical artery of the pump twin in a reversed direction into the umbilical artery of the perfused twin via an arterio-arterial anastomosis. The perfused twin's blood supply is by definition deoxygenated and results in variable degrees of deficient development of the head, heart, and upper limb structures. Two criteria seem to be necessary for the development of a TRAP sequence: (1) an arterio-arterial anastomosis and (2) a discordant development [39] or an IUFD [40] in one of monochorionic twins, which allows for reversal of blood flow. The increased burden to perfuse the parasitic twin puts the pump twin at risk for congestive heart failure and hydrops [41]. Because of the rarity of the disorder, the natural history of antenatally diagnosed cases is still poorly documented, with reported survival rates for the pump twin varying between 14% [42] and 90% [43]. Data on long-term outcome are not available, although the risk of cardiac and neurodevelopmental sequelae may be high because of vascular imbalances in utero [44,45]. Prediction of outcome of TRAP diagnosed in the early second trimester is challenging. Several parameters have been suggested to indicate poor prognosis, such as a high acardiac/pump weight ratio [46], a rapid increase in the acardiac mass [47], and small differences in the umbilical artery Doppler values [48,49]. These parameters were mostly studied in late second and third trimester, however, and do not necessary apply in the early second trimester, when spontaneous resolution and sudden death of the pump twin remain unpredictable. Early intervention is an issue, because today the diagnosis is usually made at an early stage in pregnancy. Early prophylactic intervention may preclude the technical difficulties of achieving arrest of flow in larger and often hydropic acardiac masses. Some physicians may therefore prefer to offer prophylactic, minimally invasive intervention if no spontaneous arrest of flow has occurred by 16 weeks, recognizing that the pump twin may survive without any intervention in at least 50% of cases.

For the treatment of TTTS, selective feticide has been proposed, merely to try to salvage one twin [50,51]. The rationale is that laser coagulation has such a high risk of IUFD of one twin that it acts as a selective feticide. Cord occlusion may seem to be an attractive alternative because it is technically easier to perform and may better protect the surviving twin. This approach is open for debate and necessarily leads to some difficult decisions. Not only does it pose a tremendous strain on the parents but also it may not be easy to determine which fetus will have the worst prognosis. Initially, researchers thought that the donor had the worst prognosis, especially if abnormal umbilical artery Doppler results were present, but these can normalize after the cord occlusion of the recipient's cord. Access to the donor is also technically more challenging, and recipients seem to be at higher risk of neurologic and cardiac sequelae [4,52]. The major drawback of this approach is the maximum survival rate of 50%. Because laser can salvage fetuses at all stages of the disease, advanced disease is not an indication [8,53]. In our opinion, fetoscopic laser coagulation remains the preferred first-line treatment, and selective feticide should be restricted to highly selected and exceptional cases.

Technique and outcome of selective feticide in dichorionic twins

Selective feticide in dichorionic twins is performed by intracardiac or intra-funicular injection of potassium chloride under ultrasound guidance. It is of utmost importance to ascertain that the correct fetus is terminated by identi-fication of gender differences, obvious structural anomalies, placental localiza-tions, and cord insertions. The risks of selective termination include loss of the entire pregnancy and premature delivery. The overall loss rate reported by the international selective feticide registry of 402 multiple pregnancies, including some higher-order multiple pregnancies, is 7.5%. Preterm delivery before 33 weeks' gestation occurred in 22%, with 6% delivering between 25 and 28 weeks [54]. One center with 200 selective feticides reported an overall loss rate of only 4%, with 16% of patients delivering before 32 weeks [55]. This finding underscores the importance of the procedure being performed by experienced hands. To reduce loss rates, researchers have proposed deferring selective feticide to 28 to 32 weeks' gestation, which is only an option in countries in which late termination is legal, and it may be emotionally more difficult to accept for parents and doctors. In a series on 23 dichorionic twins managed with late seletive feticide, there were no fetal losses and all patients delivered beyond 35 weeks' gestation [56].

Technique and outcome of selective feticide in monochorionic twins

For selective feticide in monochorionic multiple pregnancies, the conventional techniques of potassium chloride injection used in multichorionic pregnancies cannot be used. Minimally invasive techniques have been proposed to arrest and isolate the target twin's circulation completely and permanently [57], although all have considerably higher risks for fetal loss compared with the injection of potassium chloride.

Currently, the preferred method for selective feticide in monochorionic multiple pregnancies is cord occlusion by either laser or bipolar coagulation. The initially reported method of umbilical cord embolization using various agents is no longer recommended because of failure rates of more than 60% [58,59], probably because of incomplete vascular obliteration or migration of the toxic products to the co-twin. Fetoscopic cord ligation is already a historical technique, although it does cause immediate, complete, and permanent interruption of arterial and venous flow. Despite the fact that co-twin survival rates are more than 70% when the procedure is performed fetoscopically, it is a cumbersome technique with a high risk for PPROM [60]. In contrast, fetoscopic laser coagulation of the umbilical cord is a simple technique similar to fetoscopic coagulation of the vascular anastomoses in TTTS. It has been performed as early as 16 weeks' gestation using a double needle loaded with a 1 mm fetoscope and a 400 μm laser fiber [61]. The procedure allows optimal visual control but may fail beyond 20 weeks' gestation because of increasing size of the umbilical cord vessels [62]. Ultrasound-guided bipolar cord coagulation was introduced for selective feticide at later gestational ages. In our institution, we use laser coagulation before 21 weeks' gestation, laser with back-up bipolar between 21 and 26 weeks, and bipolar after 26 weeks [63].

The pre- and postoperative care and access method is similar to that described for laser coagulation of the vascular anastomoses in TTTS. At all times, a double set-up for fetoscopic laser and ultrasound-guided bipolar coagulation is used. The site of port insertion is chosen according to the position of the placenta, the amniotic sac of the target fetus, and its umbilical cord. Preferred entry is in the sac of the target fetus. Whenever necessary, amniodrainage or amnioinfusion with warmed Hartmann's solution at 38°C is performed to reduce or expand the working space around the target cord or to improve endoscopic vision.

Laser coagulation is performed by an Nd:YAG laser or diode laser with bare fibers of 600 μm. The cord is coagulated over a distance of 5 to 10 cm using a non-touch technique in continuous mode at 30 to 50 W (Fig. 11). Absence of flow is interrogated by color Doppler. Septostomy can be performed by laser when direct access to the target sac is not possible and laser coagulation through

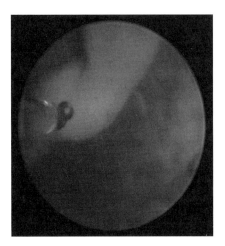

Fig. 11. Fetoscopic image of laser cord coagulation.

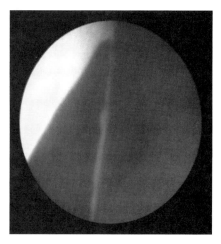

Fig. 12. Fetoscopic image of the hole in the intertwin septum after septostomy by laser.

the intertwin septum fails (Fig. 12). Bipolar coagulation is performed with a 3- or 2.4-mm forceps, according to the cord diameter. Under ultrasound guidance, a portion of the umbilical cord is grasped at the abdominal wall, its placental insertion, or any other appropriate place to ensure correct identification and enhance stability (Fig. 13). Direct contact with the placenta, fetus, or membranes is avoided. To improve visual control, a new "optical" forceps is being evaluated within the Eurofoetus project that combines the advantages of bipolar coagulation and fetoscopy. Coagulation starts at power settings of 15 W applied for approximately 15 seconds and advances with progressive increments of 2 to 5 W until turbulence and steam bubbles appear between the forceps' blades, which indicate local heat production and eventual tissue coagulation (usually between 30 and 45 W). Higher initial energy settings are avoided to prevent tissue carbonization, which may lead to the cord becoming stuck to the forceps' blades and eventual cord perforation. Confirmation of arrest of flow is performed after the forceps is freed from the umbilical cord by gentle manipulation. Even if flow is no longer visible, two additional cord segments (preferably at a site more proximal to the target fetus) are coagulated. This is an additional safety precaution, because absence of Doppler flow may be caused by temporary vasospasm rather than true vascular obliteration. To avoid later cord entanglement in mono-amniotic twins, the cord is first coagulated and then transected with laser in contact mode (Fig. 14). After completion of the procedure, amniodrainage of excessive fluid is performed before removal of the cannula. Middle cerebral artery Doppler is performed postoperatively to detect fetal anemia.

In our initial ten cases, two patients had PPROM and underwent a termination. The other eight patients delivered at a mean gestational age of 35 weeks (ie, more than 15 weeks after the procedure) [56]. Nicolini et al [64] reported their experience with 17 cases. The survival rate was 81% (13/16 survivors; one pa-

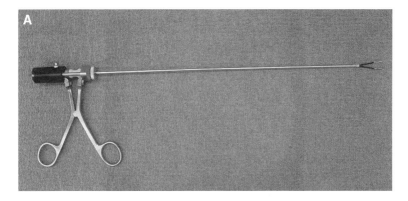

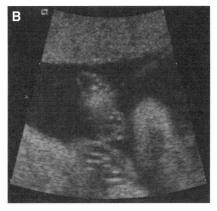

Fig. 13. (A) Reusable 2.4-mm bipolar forceps (Karl Storz, Tuttlingen, Germany). (B) Ultrasound image of the bipolar forceps grasping the umbilical cord at its placental insertion.

tient had TOP because of an abnormality diagnosed later). One fetal hemorrhage was caused by cord perforation, which may be avoided by not applying too much energy. We reported the outcome of 50 consecutive cord coagulations in complicated monochorionic multiples (including four triplets) by laser or bipolar coagulation performed between 16 and 28 weeks' gestation (mean, 21 weeks) [65]. Indications were TRAP (38%), discordant anomaly (38%), selected cases of severe TTTS (20%), and selective intrauterine growth restriction (4%). In 75% of cases, laser was used as the primary energy, but additional bipolar was necessary in approximately half of cases. Overall survival rate was 75% with normal outcome (range: 1–36 months, 63% follow-up), except for one child with mild developmental delay born after PPROM at less than 28 weeks' gestation. Persistent PPROM at less than 30 weeks occurred in 25%; cases that involved PPROM at less than 25 weeks were associated with a mortality rate of 80%. There were no serious maternal complications, except for one mild transient mirror or Ballantyne syndrome. To avoid the risks of early PPROM for the

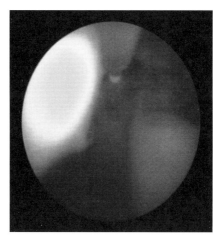

Fig. 14. Fetoscopic image of a cord transection by laser in contact mode after selective feticide in monoamniotic twins.

healthy co-twin, there is a strong argument for deferring selective feticide until after 24 weeks in highly selected cases of discordant anomaly in which the risk of IUFD is small (such as in severe discordant central nervous system, genito-urinary, or skeletal anomaly), at least in countries in which this is legally possible and when it is ethically acceptable. Bipolar coagulation can be performed using the 3-mm forceps by overstretching the blades, whereupon the forceps opens more widely to accommodate for the larger cord diameter, as showed in a consecutive series of five cases performed between 26 and 30 weeks' gestation. All deliveries occurred beyond 31 weeks (range, 31–37 weeks). All infants survived, except for one unrelated neonatal death of a child born at 36 weeks because of a complication of balloon dilatation for pulmonary stenosis [66].

Summary

Complications unique to monochorionic twins and the shared circulation have stimulated a revival of fetoscopy as a means of operating on the placenta and umbilical cord. Currently, fetoscopic laser coagulation of the vascular anasto-moses is the preferred first-line treatment for TTTS, which complicates 10% to 15% of monochorionic multiple pregnancies. Minimally invasive cord coagu-lation seems to be an effective technique for selective feticide in pregnancy with monochorionic twins complicated by discordant anomaly, severe early discordant growth, TRAP, and selected cases of TTTS. However, these procedures still have considerably higher fetal loss rates (25%) compared with selective feticide in dichorionic twins (7.5%).

Acknowledgments

The authors would like to thank the other members of the EuroTwin2Twin Consortium for setting up the group: Y. Ville (Poissy), K. Hecher (Hamburg), E. Gratacos (Barcelona), R. Vlietinck (Leuven), M. van Gemert (Amsterdam), G. Barki (Tuttlingen), K. Nicolaides (London), R. Denk (München), and C. Jackson (London).

References

[1] Caroll SGM, Soothill PW, Abdel-Fattah SA, et al. Prediction of chorionicity in twin pregnancies at 10–14 weeks of gestation. Br J Obstet Gynaecol 2002;109:182–6.

[2] Denbow ML, Cox P, Taylor M, et al. Placental angioarchitecture in monochorionic twin pregnancies: relationship to fetal growth, fetofetal transfusion syndrome, and pregnancy outcome. Am J Obstet Gynecol 2000;182:417–26.

[3] Gratacós E, Deprest J. Current experience with fetoscopy and the Eurofoetus registry for fetoscopic procedures. Eur J Obstet Gynecol Reprod Biol 2000;92:151–60.

[4] Senat MV, Deprest J, Boulvain M, et al. Endoscopic laser surgery versus serial amnioreduction for severe twin-to-twin transfusion syndrome. N Engl J Med 2004;8,351(2):136–44.

[5] Lewi L, Van Schoubroeck D, Gratacos E, et al. Monochorionic diamniotic twins: complications and management options. Curr Opin Obstet Gynecol 2003;15:177–94.

[6] Challis D, Gratacós E, Deprest J. Selective termination in monochorionic twins. J Perinat Med 1999;27:327–38.

[7] Campbell S. Opinion: twin-to-twin transfusion syndrome. Debates on the etiology, natural history and management. Ultrasound Obstet Gynecol 2000;16:210–3.

[8] Eurofoetus. Endoscopic feto-placental surgery: from animal experimentation to early human experimentation. Brussels, Belgium: European Commission, within the Biomed 2 Programme; BMH CT 4 97 2382, 1998.

[9] Deprest J, Van Schoubroeck D, Van Ballaer P, et al. Alternative access for fetoscopic Nd:YAG laser in TTS with anterior placenta. Ultrasound Obstet Gynecol 1998;12:347–52.

[10] Luks FI, Deprest JA, Vandenberghe K, et al. Fetoscopy-guided fetal endoscopy in a sheep model. J Am Coll Surg 1994;178:609–12.

[11] Quintero RA, Bornick PW, Allen MH, et al. Selective photocoagulation of communicating vessels in severe twin-twin transfusion syndrome in women with an anterior placenta. Obstet Gynecol 2001;97:477–81.

[12] Deprest J, Ville Y. Obstetric endoscopy. In: Harrison M, Evans M, Adzick NS, et al, editors. The unborn patient: the art and science of fetal therapy. Philadelphia: WB Saunders; 2000. p. 213–32.

[13] Deprest J, Van Schoubroeck D, Carreras E, et al. Operative fetoscopy. In: Evans M, Johnson M, Wapner R, editors. Prenatal diagnosis. New York: McGraw Hill; 2002.

[14] Quintero RA. Diagnostic and operative fetoscopy: technical issues. In: Quintero RA, editor. Diagnostic and operative fetoscopy. New York: Parthenon; 2002. p. 7–20.

[15] Bonati F, Perales A, Novak P, et al. Ex vivo testing of a temperature and pressure controlled amnio-irrigator for fetoscopic surgery. J Pediatr Surg 2002;37:18–24.

[16] Feldstein VA, Machin GA, Albanese CT, et al. Twin-twin transfusion syndrome: the select procedure. Fetal Diagn Ther 2000;15:257–61.

[17] Quintero RA, Comas C, Bornick PW, et al. Selective versus non-selective laser photocoagulation of placental vessels in twin-to-twin transfusion syndrome. Ultrasound Obstet Gynecol 2000; 16(3):230–6.

[18] Lewi L, Cannie M, Vandecaveye V, et al. A pilot study to assess the role of placental MR

imaging to predict placental distribution and the position of the vascular equator in twin-to-twin transfusion syndrome. Ultrasound Obstet Gynecol 2004;24(3):118, 248.

[19] Senat MV, Loizeau S, Couderc S, et al. The value of middle cerebral artery peak systolic velocity in the diagnosis of fetal anemia after intrauterine death of one monochorionic twin. Am J Obstet Gynecol 2003;189(5):1320–4.

[20] Sutcliff AG, Sebire NJ, Pigott AJ, et al. Outcome of children born after in utero laser ablation therapy for severe twin-to-twin transfusion syndrome. Br J Obstet Gynaecol 2001;108:1246–50.

[21] Lopriore E, Nagel HT, Vandenbussche FP, et al. Long-term neurodevelopmental outcome in twin-to-twin transfusion syndrome. Am J Obstet Gynecol 2003;189(5):1314–9.

[22] Quintero RA, Morales WJ, Allen M, et al. Treatment of iatrogenic previable premature rupture of membranes with intra-amniotic injection of platelets and cryoprecipitate (amniopatch): preliminary experience. Am J Obstet Gynecol 1999;181(3):744–9.

[23] Lewi L, Van Schoubroeck D, Van Ranst M, et al. Successful patching of iatrogenic rupture of the fetal membranes. Placenta 2004;25(4):352–6.

[24] Stone CA, Quinn MW, Saxby PJ. Congenital skin loss following Nd:YAG placental coagulation. Burns 1998;24:275–7.

[25] Luks F, Carr S, Tracy T. Intestinal complications associated with twin-twin transfusion syndrome after antenatal laser treatment: report of 2 cases. J Pediatr Surg 2001;36:1105–6.

[26] Scott F, Evans N. Distal gangrene in a polycythemic recipient fetus in twin-twin transfusion. Obstet Gynecol 1995;86:677–9.

[27] Banek CS, Hecher K, Hackeloer BJ, et al. Long-term neurodevelopmental outcome after intrauterine laser treatment for severe twin-twin transfusion syndrome. Am J Obstet Gynecol 2003;188(4):876–80.

[28] Hecher K, Diehl W, Zikulnig L, et al. Endoscopic laser coagulation of placental anastomoses in 200 pregnancies with severe mid-trimester twin-to-twin transfusion syndrome. Eur J Obstet Gynecol Reprod Biol 2000;92(1):135–40.

[29] Lewi L, Vandenberghe G, Deprest J. Fertility and pregnancy outcome after fetoscopic surgery. Am J Obstet Gynecol 2003;S189(6):S597.

[30] Baldwin VJ. Anomalous development in twins. In: Baldwin VJ, editor. Pathology of multiple pregnancies. New York: Springer-Verlag; 1994. p. 169–97.

[31] Bryan E, Little J. Congenital anomalies in twins. Baillieres Clin Obstet Gynecol 1987;1: 697–721.

[32] Heydanus R, Santema JG, Steward PA, et al. Preterm delivery rate and fetal outcome in structurally affected twin pregnancies: a retrospective matched control study. Prenat Diagn 1993;13(3):155–62.

[33] Nieuwint A, Van Zalen-Sprock R, Hummel P, et al. Identical twins with normal karyotypes. Prenat Diagn 1999;19(1):72–6.

[34] Lewi L, Van Schoubroeck D, Gloning K-P, et al. Selective feticide by cord occlusion in four sets of heterokaryotypic monochorionic twins. J Soc Gynecol Investig 2003;10(Suppl):405.

[35] Bajoria R, Wee LY, Anwar S, et al. Outcome of twin pregnancies complicated by single intrauterine death in relation to vascular anatomy of the monochorionic placenta. Hum Reprod 1999;14(8):2124–30.

[36] Nicolini U, Poblete A. Single intrauterine death in monochorionic twins pregnancies. Ultrasound Obstet Gynecol 1999;14:297–301.

[37] Adegbite AL, Castille S, Ward S, et al. Neuromorbidity in preterm twins in relation to chorionicity and discordant birth weight. Am J Obstet Gynecol 2004;190(1):156–63.

[38] Gratacos E, Carreras E, Becker J, et al. Prevalence of neurological damage in monochorionic twins with selective intrauterine growth restriction and intermittent absent or reversed end-diastolic umbilical artery flow. Ultrasound Obstet Gynecol 2004;24(2):159–63.

[39] Van Allen MI, Smith DW, Shephard TH. Twin reversed arterial perfusion (TRAP) sequence: a study of 14 twin pregnancies with acardiacus. Semin Perinatol 1983;7:285–93.

[40] Gembruch U, Viski S, Bagamery K, et al. Twin reversed arterial perfusion sequence in twin-to-twin transfusion syndrome after the death of the donor co-twin in the second trimester. Ultrasound Obstet Gynecol 2001;17:153–6.

[41] Gilliam DL, Hendricks CH. Holoacardius: review of literature and case report. Obstet Gynecol 1953;2:647–53.

[42] Sogaard K, Skibsted L, Brocks V. Acardiac twins: pathophysiology, diagnosis, outcome and treatment. Six cases and review of the literature. Fetal Diagn Ther 1999;14(1):53–9.

[43] Sullivan AE, Varner MW, Ball RH, et al. The management of acardiac twins: a conservative approach. Am J Obstet Gynecol 2003;189(5):1310–3.

[44] Chandra S, Crane JM, Young DC, et al. Acardiac twin pregnancy with neonatal resolution of donor twin cardiomyopathy. Obstet Gynecol 2000;96(5 Pt 2):820–1.

[45] Kosno-Kruszewska E, Deregowski K, Schmidt-Sidor B, et al. Neuropathological and anatomo-pathological analyses of acardiac and "normal" siblings in an acardiac-twin pregnancy. Folia Neuropathol 2003;41(2):103–9.

[46] Moore TR, Gale S, Benirschke K. Perinatal outcome of forty-nine pregnancies complicated by acardiac twinning. Am J Obstet Gynecol 1990;163(3):907–12.

[47] Brassard M, Fouron JC, Leduc L, et al. Prognostic markers in twin pregnancies with an acardiac fetus. Obstet Gynecol 1999;94(3):409–14.

[48] Sherer DM, Armstrong B, Shah YG, et al. Prenatal sonographic diagnosis, Doppler velo-cimetric umbilical cord studies, and subsequent management of an acardiac twin pregnancy. Obstet Gynecol 1989;74:472–5.

[49] Dashe JS, Fernandez CO, Twickler DM. Utility of Doppler velocimetry in predicting outcome in twin reversed-arterial perfusion sequence. Am J Obstet Gynecol 2001;185(1):135–9.

[50] Mahone PR, Sherer DM, Abramowicz JS, et al. Twin transfusion syndrome: rapid develop-ment of severe hydrops of the donor following selective fetocide of the recipient. Am J Obstet Gynecol 1993;169:166–8.

[51] Taylor MJ, Shalev E, Tanawattanacharoen S, et al. Ultrasound-guided umbilical cord occlusion using bipolar diathermy for Stage III/IV twin-twin transfusion syndrome. Prenat Diagn 2002;22(1):70–6.

[52] Zosmer N, Bajoria R, Weiner E, et al. Clinical and echocardiographic features of in utero cardiac dysfunction in the recipient twin in twin-twin transfusion syndrome. Br Heart J 1994;72:74–9.

[53] Quintero RA, Comas C, Bornick PW, et al. Selective versus non-selective laser photocoagu-lation of placental vessels in twin-to-twin transfusion syndrome. Ultrasound Obstet Gynecol 2000;16:230–6.

[54] Evans MI, Goldberg JD, Horenstein J, et al. Selective termination for structural, chromosomal, and mendelian anomalies: international experience. Am J Obstet Gynecol 1999;181(4):893–7.

[55] Eddleman KA, Stone JL, Lynch L, et al. Selective termination of anomalous fetuses in multifetal pregnancies: two hundred cases at a single center. Am J Obstet Gynecol 2002;187(5):1168–72.

[56] Deprest JA, Audibert F, Van Schoubroeck D, et al. Bipolar coagulation of the umbilical cord in complicated monochorionic twin pregnancy. Am J Obstet Gynecol 2000;182(2):340–5.

[57] Challis D, Gratacós E, Deprest J. Selective termination in monochorionic twins. J Perinat Med 1999;27:327–38.

[58] Denbow ML, Overton TG, Duncan KR, et al. High failure rate of umbilical vessel occlusion by ultrasound guided injection of absolute alcohol or enbucrilate gel. Prenat Diagn 1999;19: 527–32.

[59] Challis D, Gratacós E, Deprest J. Selective termination in monochorionic twins. J Perinat Med 1999;27:327–38.

[60] Deprest JA, Evrard VA, Van Ballaer PP, et al. Experience with fetoscopic cord ligation. Eur J Obstet Gynecol Reprod Biol 1998;81:157–64.

[61] Hecher K, Hackeloer BJ, Ville Y. Umbilical cord coagulation by operative microendoscopy at 16 weeks' gestation in an acardiac twin. Ultrasound Obstet Gynecol 1997;10(2):130–2.

[62] Ville Y, Hyett JA, Vandenbussche FP, et al. Endoscopic laser coagulation of umbilical cord vessels in twin reversed arterial perfusion sequence. Ultrasound Obstet Gynecol 1994;4(5): 396–8.

[63] Ville Y. Selective feticide in monochorionic pregnancies: toys for the boys or standard of care? Ultrasound Obstet Gynecol 2003;22(5):448–50.

[64] Nicolini U, Poblete A, Boschetto C, et al. Complicated monochorionic twin pregnancies: experience with bipolar cord coagulation. Am J Obstet Gynecol 2000;185:703–7.

[65] Lewi L, Gratacos E, Van Schoubroeck D, et al. 50 consecutive cord coagulations in monochorionic multiplets [abstract 21]. Am J Obstet Gynecol 2003;187(6):S61.

[66] Deprest J, Van Schoubroeck D, Senat M-V, et al. Cord coagulation in monochorionic multiplets late in gestation. Am J Obstet Gynecol 2003;S189(6):S612.

ELSEVIER
SAUNDERS

Obstet Gynecol Clin N Am
32 (2005) 127–139

OBSTETRICS AND
GYNECOLOGY
CLINICS
OF NORTH AMERICA

En Route to an "Instant Family": Psychosocial Considerations

Liora Baor, MSW[a],*, Isaac Blickstein, MD[b]

[a]Faculty of Social Sciences, School of Social Work, Bar-Ilan University, Ramat-Gan 52900, Israel
[b]Department of Obstetrics and Gynecology, Kaplan Medical Center, Rehovot 76100, Israel

A young couple calls a travel agent and asks for the best deal for their ultimate honeymoon vacation. The agent suggests two possibilities for starting the wonderful vacation: (1) a flight with "Vital Airlines," a company with a 1:10,000 chance of crashing and (2) a flight with "Mortal Airlines," a company with a 1:1,000 chance to crash. Which airline will the couple choose? The answer—and the analogy—are clear.

Assisted reproductive technology (ART) may produce a serious side effect— multiple pregnancy—that is a complication frequently either overlooked or underappreciated by an infertile couple. Multiple births are associated with adverse perinatal outcomes: 58.2% of twins compared with 10.4% of singletons are delivered preterm (< 37 weeks' gestation), and 55.4% of twins compared with 6.1% of singletons are low birth weight (< 2500 g) [1]. 11.9% of twins compared with 1.6% of singletons are delivered very preterm (< 32 weeks' gestation), and 10.2% of twins compared with 1.1% of singletons are very low birth weight (< 1500 g) [1]. These figures are even more alarming in triplets and higher-order multiples. Not surprisingly, studies on perinatal outcomes after in vitro fertilization (IVF) indicate that multiple pregnancies are associated with a 7-fold higher rate of neonatal mortality in twins and more than 20-fold higher rate in triplets and higher-order births [2]. Population-based studies also indicate long-term consequences: three- to sixfold higher incidence of cerebral palsy in twins compared with singletons and more than a tenfold higher incidence

This article was adapted from Baor L, Blickstein I. The journey from infertility to parenting multiples: a dream come true? Int J Fertil Womens Med; in press.

* Corresponding author.
E-mail address: lbaor@netvision.net.il (L. Baor).

of cerebral palsy in triplets [3]. Box 1 shows the perinatal risks that are specifically increased in multiple pregnancies compared with singletons.

Regardless of these potential adverse outcomes, increasing numbers of couples are choosing ART as means of conception. The results of this trend are reflected in the increased numbers of multiple births worldwide. Most countries report a 20% to 30% incidence of multiple births after ART leading to an increased incidence of multiples in the general population. For example, the twin birth rate in the United States has increased steadily since 1980 to 31.1 twins per 1000 total live births in 2002. The rate has climbed 38% since 1990 (22.6 per 1000), and 65% since 1980 (18.9 per 1000) [1].

Box 1. Complications that are more frequently encountered in multiple pregnancies

Maternal

Hypertensive disorders

Pre-eclamptic toxemia (HELP syndrome, acute fatty liver)
Pregnancy-induced hypertension
Chronic hypertension
Eclampsia

Anemia
Gestational diabetes mellitus (?)
Premature contractions and labor

Complications associated with tocolysis

Delivery-associated complications

Cesarean section
Operative delivery
Premature rupture of membranes
Postpartum endometritis
Placental abruption

Fetal-neonatal

Malformations
Monozygosity-related conditions
Preterm birth
Growth aberrations

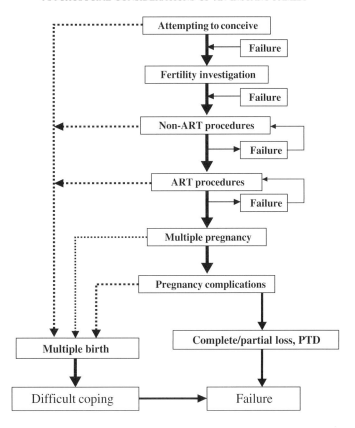

Fig. 1. The route from infertility to multiple birth. Dotted and solid lines show successful and failures, respectively.

This article discusses the difficult route of patients who undergo ART who wish to complete their family instantly by having a multiple pregnancy. We discuss the psychosocial aspects of the various steps en route. It seems that most of the multiple pregnancy–related problems are not adequately anticipated by infertile patients and lead to psychosocial distress that has major implications on interpersonal and intrapersonal aspects. Fig. 1 is a simplified description of the long and winding road from being infertile to being parents of multiples.

Parenting motives

Motives for parenthood are based on a mixture of cultural-societal and interpersonal values. Historically, Western cultures idealized women who became mothers, the so-called "myth of motherhood," but the mandatory nature of parenthood was extended to include the roles of fathers too. Traditional fertility norms, whereby married couples should want to reproduce, continue to be accepted widely in the Western world [4], and in contemporary society, parenthood is perceived as the central developmental task of midlife. Societal and cultural norms require that a "worthwhile person" engage in behaviors that show normalcy and responsibility, such as bearing and raising children [5]. The notion that femininity is quasi-synonymous with motherhood excludes and deprives childless women of the most central elements of gender identity and personal integrity [4]. It should be noted, however, that the current American society values individualistic and hedonistic norms that reflect in higher rates of voluntarily childless couples.

From a personal view, the main reasons for wanting a child include the desire to give and receive love, have primary group ties and affection, enjoy stimulation and fun, and experience happiness followed by well-being, continuity, and enjoyment of children [6].

In paternalistic societies, procreation norms are imperative. For example, in Israel, where childbirth is considered among the highest personal priorities, one's entire life may center on procreation. This high social value of fertility is reflected in public and health care policies, whereby the Israeli Health Insurance Law provides for an unlimited number of IVF or other relevant infertility treatments until two children are born. In such circumstances, being childless is an unbearable stigma and there is little chance of being socially accepted as a single, rich, and childless individual, as is often the case in the United States [7].

Young adults who assume that they will bear and raise children also may presume erroneously that fertility is granted. In such cases, contraception is used to postpone childbirth until certain milestones in education and career are achieved. When the time for a pregnancy arrives, however, some couples may find that parenthood is beyond their control and out of their reach.

In a society in which fertility is linked with adulthood and sexuality, infertility can affect one's self-esteem, competence, adequacy, and efficacy deeply [8,9]. For societies in which childbearing is a social and cultural imperative, childless couples may feel different and deprived and become determined to seek a solution. In this respect, ART is considered the ultimate salvation of the current infertile generation, because ART technically bypasses the infertility problem and helps a couple to fulfill their goals within the sociocultural frame of their life.

ART procedures are highly stressful and demand diverse personal coping resources for men and women [10]. Despite difficulties, ART is inevitable for two main reasons. First, patients cannot ignore the availability and efficacy of a technology to solve most infertility problems, and second, the goal of parenthood justifies every available means, including ART.

Stresses associated with infertility

Infertility potentially may lead to significant negative consequences, especially when treatment fails. The diagnosis and treatment of infertility may

---

Box 2. Losses that accompany infertility

Loss of relationships

With spouse
With social network

Loss of health

Impaired body image

Loss of prestige
Loss of self-esteem
Loss of confidence and control

Control of one's own life
Control of future

Loss of security

Financially
Professionally

Loss of hope

---

have deleterious effects on women and men's subjective well-being. These apparently healthy couples suddenly become "patients" whose most intimate elements of life begin to revolve around a physician's scheme. The prime focus on conception affects a couple's self-esteem, confidence, health, close relationship, security, and hope (Box 2). Prevalent emotional responses include grief, depression, anger, guilt, shock or denial, and anxiety [11,12].

Effects on self-esteem

Self-esteem is defined as "the extent which one prizes, values, approves, or likes oneself" [13]. For some couples, failure to conceive is likely to diminish their own pride, an effect that may be accentuated by daily self-reminders of the inability to accomplish their own expectations. Feelings of failure and inadequacy are not limited to reproductive dysfunction; rather, such reactions may diminish the sense of femininity or masculinity and impair body image and self-esteem [12].

Effects on social relationships

Although mutual support seems a reasonable expectation, infertile couples often express negative effects and disapproval because of shared stresses [14]. The couple may suffer loss of closeness and experience increased isolation, and the end of a relationship may be either an actual or an unspoken threat [12]. Some individuals report increased anger, hostility, or resentment toward their spouse as a result of lack of emotional support or feeling that the other partner is not equally committed to parenthood [12]. In contrast, there is evidence of increased closeness, love, and support among couples who undergo infertility treatment [8,11].

In addition to potential impairment in spousal relationships, social relationships with "significant others" (a term used to describe socially meaningful individuals) also may diminish. Couples report feeling socially unworthy or isolated and report feelings of jealousy, rivalry, resentment, and envy toward people who have children. Such feelings are sometimes directed toward other family members with children who are biologically similar [8,10]. Many couples are unwilling to discuss openly and share their infertility problems with others because of the embarrassment and discomfort associated with sexual issues, a situation that further isolates an involuntary childless couple [14].

Effects on internal control

In this sense, the term "control" refers to an individual's beliefs about who or what determines outcome of one's life [15]. Self-directed individuals who seem to be in control of their lives may become distressed by the infertility experience. Because ART procedures demand high commitment and adherence, life may seem to revolve around physicians' appointments in the sense that infertility treatments seem to control life rather than the other way round. Because of this inevitable side effect, some couples feel loss of control over their ability to plan for the future [12].

Because the course of treatment often requires scheduled sexual intercourse, infertility treatment also challenges sexual spontaneity, and the need to have "sex on demand" often makes it a chore rather than a pleasure. The constant intrusion into the most intimate aspects of life can—in men and women—reduce the feeling of being desired and lead to avoidance of spontaneous sexual activity and failure to function on demand, which ultimately may cause sexual dissatisfaction [12,16]. The uncomfortable and sometimes unsuccessful diagnostic and medical procedures involved with infertility may compel couples to believe that their bodies are impaired. Individuals who pride themselves on taking care of their bodies may find the diagnosis of infertility incompatible with their previous perception of well-being.

Effects on financial security

Couples may become stressful and insecure about the financial burden caused by repeated appointments, interventions, and medications. Because it is impossible to predict how many cycles are required to conceive in a given case, couples may invest almost anything in their pursuit for a baby. According to estimates from the European Society of Human Reproduction and Embryology, the average cost per cycle of IVF and Intracytoplasmic sperm injection (ICSI) in 2002 would be US$9547 in the United States and US$3518 in 25 other countries. The cost to the individual couple ranges from 10% of the annual household expenditures in European countries to 25% in Canada and the United States [17]. The dictated schedule of infertility treatments often affects job security and promotion. Some individuals turn down promotions, relocation, or career changes to keep in touch with physicians and maintain the liberty to miss work for medical appointments [12].

On a deeper level, loss of security regarding fairness and predictability of life commonly exists. Couples may expend great effort to determine why they are infertile and how they could have prevented it. They often fear that if they could be afflicted by infertility, they could be afflicted with everything else [11].

Psychological reactions to failure of in vitro fertilization

For many couples, IVF is the last resort to having their "own" child. When IVF fails (as is the case in 60% to 80% of treatment cycles), a couple eventually acknowledges being infertile and may begin to mourn the child who was never conceived. Women also may mourn the loss of opportunity to experience pregnancy, delivery, and nursing. Men and women may mourn the lost chance to perpetuate their genes and gain social acceptance by the society that values pregnancy and parenting [18]. After an unsuccessful IVF treatment, couples may experience severe stress, disappointment, sadness, anger, and depression, all of which are more evident in women than men [19]. In another study, women who underwent IVF were more depressed, scored lower on self-confidence, and had lower self-esteem than women who did not undergo the treatment [20]. Slade et al [21] found that 6 months after completing three unsuccessful IVF cycles, couples were emotionally more distressed and showed poorer marital and sexual adjustment than couples who achieved a pregnancy.

The desire for multiples

Infertile patients often ignore the real risks of multiple pregnancy and births and express a wish for multiples [22]. Murdoch [23] evaluated 150 replies to a questionnaire regarding the ideal outcome of IVF treatment. Of the respondents, 69% considered a multiple pregnancy as an ideal outcome, and the increased duration of infertility significantly contributed to this desire for multiples [22,23]. In the study by Child et al [24], patients who underwent IVF were asked to state the desired number of babies with their next fertility treatment. The authors reported that 41% of patients considered a multiple pregnancy an ideal outcome. Ryan et al [25] also studied the desired outcome of IVF treatment, with a possible reply of having one to as many as four or more babies. In this sample, 20.3% of the patients listed a multiple birth as the most desired outcome, most of whom (94%) ranked twins as their most desired outcome.

The dream of two or three children as an outcome of one pregnancy does not include handicapped children, nor does it include an unhealthy mother—both of which are potential untoward outcomes of a multiple pregnancy and birth. When patients are aware of these risks, however, the enthusiasm for a multiple birth decreases. In the study by Grobman et al [26], the appreciation of increased fetal risks associated with a multiple pregnancy significantly contributed to a decreased desire for such an outcome. More recently, Pinborg et al [27] studied the expectation of singletons versus twins as a desired outcome in mothers of twins and singletons (aged 4–5 years) who were conceived either with or without IVF. Among mothers of twins conceived with IVF, 85% preferred twins for their first pregnancy, compared with 62% of mothers of singletons or babies conceived without IVF. Conversely, patients who recognize the increased risks of a multiple pregnancy are significantly less likely to wish to have twins.

The results of these studies imply a correlation between the duration of infertility and the wish to have a multiple pregnancy or even higher-order multiples, which suggests that individuals who confronted unsuccessful infertility treatments for many years consider themselves fortunate to have two or even three babies at once [22–27]. As a result, clinicians who are aware of the pathologies involved with multiple pregnancy and birth should not be surprised at a patient's desperate wish for an "instant family." Only a few couples consider the practical, financial, and emotional stresses that often result from having and raising multiple children. Most twin mothers nevertheless accept the potential risk of adverse outcomes and the social and physical strains involved with infertility treatment [28].

Pregnancy after in vitro fertilization

Several studies suggested that women who undergo IVF have higher rates of anxiety related to their "premium" pregnancy than women who do not undergo the procedure [29]. Women who underwent IVF expressed more anxiety about the well-being of their unborn babies and about damage to the babies during childbirth [30]. In this context, a multiple pregnancy may be more physically and emotionally stressful than a singleton pregnancy because of increased bodily discomfort, more frequent monitoring, and more obstetric interventions. The potential risks of complications in pregnancies after infertility treatments add to the stress that is already present [31]. Families that never envision the realities of parenting multiples may experience difficult adjustment to the new situation once pregnancy is over [32].

The challenge of parenting preterm multiples

Parents who were involved with IVF and who underwent a long and exhausting journey toward parenthood while expecting their "perfect" child to be born would consider the preterm birth of their multiples a great crisis. These parents may experience guilt and stress as if they were responsible for this untoward outcome [33]. Mothers of preterm infants experience higher levels of psychological distress during the neonatal period compared with mothers of full-term infants, with depression and anxiety being noted at the time of discharge from hospital [34]. In a study on the effect of infants' maturity, 91% of the parents of preterm infants felt unprepared for caring for their infants after hospital discharge, compared with 50% of parents of full-term infants [33]. Parental burdens related to caring for preterm infants depend on the severity of neonatal complications, which make the already difficult daily tasks even more time consuming [35]. Caring for two or more preterm infants or a child (or children) with special needs increases the difficulty of caring for other children of the same age who have different needs [36]. In the case of cerebral palsy, in which twins look different, the special status of having or being a twin is particularly lost. In such circumstances, the parents—and often the affected child—have a constant reminder in the unaffected child of how they might—and should—have been.

Unrealistic expectations of parents for children who were conceived with IVF can add stress that endangers the adjustment to parenthood of multiples [37]. When the children do not meet these expectations, mainly in the case of preterm birth and its sequelae, adjustment to parenthood and the important parent–child interactions are further delayed [38,39]. During infancy, parents of preterm infants are less responsive to their cues compared with parents of term infants [40]. It is possible that these parental stresses reflect in increased child abuse and neglect, consequences that were described among infants who were born preterm or suffered significant neonatal illness [41].

Perinatal death

The risk of stillbirth and neonatal death in twins is more than two and five times higher, respectively, than for singletons. For parents, the thought of carrying a live fetus for many weeks along with its dead co-twin can be disturbing. On the other hand, grieving may be delayed because the dead fetus was not aborted and its death is somehow denied [42]. After delivery, parents may be confused by the apparently contradictory feelings of rejoicing in the new life and simultaneously grieving for the dead co-twin. Complex bereavement behavior of parents results in idealization of the dead twin and positive alienation from the survivor [42].

Multifetal pregnancy reduction

The great paradox of multifetal pregnancy reduction is that couples who were desperately trying to conceive are obliged to consider termination of some embryos to allow the others to survive. The fear that all fetuses would be lost after intervention also cannot be dismissed [43]. The entire spectrum of the formidable psychosocial effects of this procedure has not been evaluated completely. However, the available data indicate that most women report guilt and mixed feelings when faced with the dilemma of multifetal pregnancy reduction [43–46]. A psychoanalytic perspective suggests that women who underwent the procedure were already vulnerable to lowered self-esteem related to their infertility, and they perceived multifetal pregnancy reduction as a "final justice" and a difficult ordeal [47].

Negative feelings are pervasive during and after multifetal pregnancy reduction. Some women use the term "murder" to describe the intervention and express guilt that they "sacrificed" one (or more) embryo to save the others [44,47]. Negative feelings are still expressed after delivery, mainly in the form of guilt and grief for the lost child. The surviving children are living reminders of the loss of the others [45]. Several investigators noted that mothers have fantasies of punishment or need forgiveness for their decision [45,47,48].

Although these negative feelings decrease with time in most mothers [48], some women report persistent dysphoric feelings, lingering sadness, and feelings of guilt [49]. Despite these grave symptoms, the initial emotional conflicts seem to have no deleterious effects on mother–child bonding [50].

Summary

The route from infertility to parenting multiples through an at-risk pregnancy is long and exhausting. For these emotionally and physically depleted couples, parenting multiples may be challenging and demanding. This wearing journey is not over with delivery of the multiples. Pregnancies further complicated by preterm birth, as is the case with many multiple pregnancies, may challenge new parents with highly demanding parental tasks, leading to higher levels of parenting stress. Couples who are unable to meet the wishful goal of having a healthy full-term pregnancy experience more stress and may question the blessings of ART.

An important issue that is discussed inadequately in the literature is the probable relationship between the wish for an instant family and the cost, in terms of money and the complexity of infertility treatment. It may well be that the wish for twins or even triplets is the logical reaction of couples who have no financial resources or are too physically and emotionally drained to undergo more treatments for a second child. Although no one is in a position to recommend that infertile couples avoid ART because of the increased risk of an untoward outcome, it is essential to acknowledge that the wish for an "instant family" by expecting or even demanding that ART provide a multiple pregnancy is basically incorrect. Physicians should provide couples with comprehensive information to enable them to make more realistic decisions.

Acknowledgments

The authors acknowledge with thanks the assistance of Prof. Louis G Keith for his valuable comments.

References

[1] Martin JA, Hamilton BE, Sutton PD, et al. Births: final data for 2002. Nat Vital Stat Rep 2003; 17;52(10):1–113.

[2] Wang JX, Norman RJ, Kristiansson P. The effect of various infertility treatments on the risk of preterm birth. Hum Reprod 2002;17(4):945–9.

[3] Blickstein I. Cerebral palsy in multifetal pregnancies. Dev Med Child Neurol 2002;44(5): 352–5.

[4] Miall CE. The stigma of involuntary childlessness. Soc Probl 1986;33:268–82.

[5] Tulandi T, Bull R, Cook R, et al. Regrettable pregnancy after infertility. Infertility 1981; 4(4):321–6.

[6] Langdrige D, Connoly K, Sheeran P. Reasons for wanting a child: a network analytic study. J Reprod Infant Psychol 2000;18(4):321–38.

[7] Remennick L. Childless in the land of imperative motherhood: stigma and coping among infertile Israeli women. Sex Roles 2000;43(11–12):821–41.

[8] Mazor MD. Emotional reactions to infertility. In: Mazor MD, Simons HF, editors. Infertility: medical, emotional, and social considerations. New York: Human Sciences Press; 1984.

[9] Cook E. Characteristics of the biopsychosocial crisis of infertility. Journal of Counseling and Development 1987;65:465–70.

[10] Dunkle-Schetter C, Lobel M. Psychological reaction to infertility. In: Stanton A, Dunkle-Schetter C, editors. Infertility: perspectives from stress and coping research. New York: Plenum Press; 1991. p. 29–57.

[11] Menning BE. The emotional needs of infertile couples. Fertil Steril 1980;34(4):313–9.

[12] Mahlstedt PP. The psychological component of infertility. Fertil Steril 1985;43(3):335–46.

[13] Blascovitch J, Tomaka J. Measures of self esteem. In: Robinson JP, Shaver PR, Wrightsman LS, editors. Measures of personality and psychological attitudes. New York: Academic Press; 1991. p. 115–60.

[14] Abbey A, Andrews FM, Halman LJ. The importance of social relationships for infertile couple's well-being. In: Stanton A, Dunkle-Schetter C, editors. Infertility: perspectives from stress and coping research. New York: Plenum Press; 1991. p. 61–86.

[15] Langer EJ. The psychology of control. Beverly Hills (CA): Sage; 1983.

[16] Abbey A. Adjusting to infertility. In: Harvey JH, Miller ED, editors. Loss and trauma: general and close relationship perspective. Philadelphia (PA): Burner-Routledge; 2000. p. 331–44.

[17] Collins JA. An international survey of the health economics of IVF and ICSI. Hum Reprod Update 2002;8(3):265–77.

[18] Keye WR. Psychosexual responses to infertility. Clin Obstet Gynecol 1984;27(3):760–6.

[19] Leiblum SR, Kemmann E, Lane MK. The psychological concomitants of in vitro fertilization. J Psychosom Obstet Gynaecol 1987;6:165–78.

[20] Hynes GJ, Callan VJ, Terry DJ, et al. The psychological well-being of infertile women after a failed IVF attempt: the effects of coping. Br J Med Psychol 1992;65(pt 3):269–78.

[21] Slade P, Emery J, Lieberman BA. A prospective longitudinal study of emotions and relationships in in vitro fertilization treatment. Hum Reprod 1997;12(1):183–90.

[22] Gleicher N, Campbell DP, Chan CL, et al. The desire for multiple births in couples with infertility problems contradicts present practice patterns. Hum Reprod 1995;10(5):1079–84.

[23] Murdoch A. Triplets and embryo transfer policy. Hum Reprod 1997;12:88–92.

[24] Child TJ, Henderson AM, Tan SL. The desire for multiple pregnancy in male and female infertility patients. Hum Reprod 2004;19(3):558–61.

[25] Ryan GL, Zhang SH, Dokras A, et al. The desire of infertile patients for multiple births. Fertil Steril 2004;81(3):500–4.

[26] Grobman WA, Milad MP, Stout J, et al. Patient perceptions of multiple gestations: an assessment of knowledge and risk aversion. Am J Obstet Gynecol 2001;185(4):920–4.

[27] Pinborg A, Loft A, Schmidt L, et al. Attitudes of IVF/ICSI twin mothers towards twins and single embryo transfer. Hum Reprod 2003;18(3):621–7.

[28] Bryan E, Denton J. The work of multiple birth foundation. J Assist Reprod Genet 2001;18(1):8–10.

[29] McMahon CA, Ungerer JA, Beaurepaire J, et al. Psychosocial outcomes for parents and children after in vitro fertilization: a review. J Reprod Infant Psychol 1995;13(10):1–16.

[30] McMahon CA, Ungerer JA, Beaurepaire J, et al. Anxiety during pregnancy and fetal attachment after in vitro fertilization conception. Hum Reprod 1997;12(1):176–82.

[31] Raoul-Duval A, Bertrand-Servais M, Frydman R. Comparative prospective study of the psychological development of children born by in vitro fertilization and their mothers. J Psychosom Obstet Gynaecol 1993;14(2):117–26.

[32] Golombok S, Cook R, Bish A, et al. Families created by the new reproductive technologies: quality of parenting and social and emotional development of the children. Child Dev 1995;66(2):285–98.

[33] Easterbrook MA. Effects of infant risk status on the transition to parenthood. In: Michaels GY, Goldberg WA, editors. The transition to parenthood: current theory and practice. New York: Cambridge University Press; 1988. p. 176–208.

[34] Pederson DR, Bento S, Chance GW, et al. Maternal emotional responses to preterm birth. Am J Orthopsychiatry 1987;57(1):15–21.

[35] Lee SK, Penner PL, Cox MC. Impact of very low birth weight infants on the family and its relationship to parental attitudes. Pediatrics 1991;88(1):105–9.

[36] Bryan E. The disabled twin. In: Bryan E, editor. Twins and higher multiple births: a guide to their nature and nurture. London: Edward Arnold; 1992. p. 165–70.

[37] Belsky J, Ward MJ, Rovine M. Parental expectations, postnatal experience and the transition to parenthood. In: Ashmore RD, Brodzinsky DM, editors. Thinking about the family: views of parents and children. Hillsdale (NJ): Lawrence Erlbaum Associates; 1986. p. 119–45.

[38] Mushin D, Spensley J, Barreda-Hanson M. Children of IVF. Clin Gynecol 1985;12(4):865–76.

[39] Belsky J. Transition to parenthood. Med Aspects Hum Sex 1986;20:56–9.

[40] Baor L, Bar-David J, Blickstein I. Psychological resource depletion in parents of twins after assisted reproduction versus spontaneous conception. Int J Fertil Womens Med 2004;49(1):13–24.

[41] Harrison MJ, Magill-Evance J. Mother and father interactions over the first year with term and preterm infants. Res Nurs Health 1996;19(6):451–9.

[42] Bryan EM. The death of a twin. In: Sandbank AC, editor. Twin and triplet psychology. London: Routhledge; 1999. p. 186–200.

[43] McKinney M, Downey J, Timor-Tritsch I. The psychological effects of multifetal pregnancy reduction. Fertil Steril 1995;64(1):51–61.

[44] Bergh C, Moller A, Nilsson L, et al. Obstetric outcome and psychological follow-up of pregnancies after embryo reduction. Hum Reprod 1999;14(8):2170–5.

[45] Maifeld M, Hahn S, Titler MG, et al. Decision making regarding multifetal reduction. J Obstet Gynecol Neonatal Nurs 2003;32(3):357–69.

[46] Bryan E. Loss in higher multiple pregnancy and multifetal pregnancy reduction. Twin Res 2002;5(3):169–74.

[47] McKinney M, Leary K. Integrating quantitative and qualitative methods to study multifetal pregnancy reduction. Womens Health 1999;8(2):259–68.

[48] Garel M, Stark C, Blondel B, et al. Psychological reactions after multifetal pregnancy reduction: a 2-year follow-up study. Hum Reprod 1997;12(3):617–22.

[49] Schreiner-Engel P, Walther VN, Mindes J, et al. First-trimester multifetal pregnancy reduction: acute and persistent psychological reactions. Am J Obstet Gynecol 1995;172(2 pt1):541–7.

[50] Kanhai HH, De Haan M, Van Zanten LA, et al. Follow-up of pregnancies, infants, and families after multifetal pregnancy reduction. Fertil Steril 1994;62(5):955–9.

ELSEVIER
SAUNDERS

Obstet Gynecol Clin N Am
32 (2005) 141–143

OBSTETRICS AND
GYNECOLOGY
CLINICS
OF NORTH AMERICA

Index

Note: Page numbers of article titles are in **boldface** type.

0889-8545/05/$ – see front matter © 2005 Elsevier Inc. All rights reserved.
doi:10.1016/S0889-8545(04)00145-7

obgyn.theclinics.com

Changing Your Address?

Make sure your subscription changes too! When you notify us of your new address, you can help make our job easier by including an exact copy of your Clinics label number with your old address (see illustration below.) This number identifies you to our computer system and will speed the processing of your address change. Please be sure this label number accompanies your old address and your corrected address—you can send an old Clinics label with your number on it or just copy it exactly and send it to the address listed below.

We appreciate your help in our attempt to give you continuous coverage. Thank you.

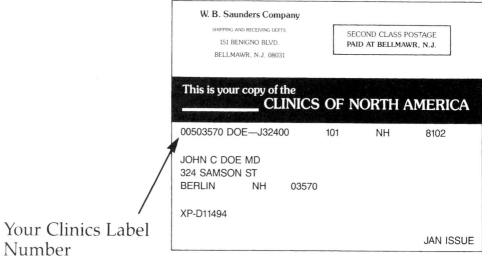

Your Clinics Label Number
Copy it exactly or send your label
along with your address to:
W.B. Saunders Company, Customer Service
Orlando, FL 32887-4800
Call Toll Free 1-800-654-2452

Please allow four to six weeks for delivery of new subscriptions and for processing address changes.

Order your subscription today. Simply complete and detach this card and drop it in the mail to receive the best clinical information in your field.

Please Print:

Name _____

Address _____

City _____ State _____ ZIP _____

Method of Payment

❏ Check (payable to **Elsevier**; add the applicable sales tax for your area)

❏ VISA　　❏ MasterCard　　❏ AmEx　　❏ Bill me

Card number _____ Exp. date _____

Signature _____

Staple this to your purchase order to expedite delivery

Adolescent Medicine Clinics
❏ Individual　$95
❏ Institutions　$133
❏ *In-training　$48

Anesthesiology
❏ Individual　$175
❏ Institutions　$270
❏ *In-training　$88

Cardiology
❏ Individual　$170
❏ Institutions　$266
❏ *In-training　$85

Chest Medicine
❏ Individual　$185
❏ Institutions　$285

Child and Adolescent Psychiatry
❏ Individual　$175
❏ Institutions　$265
❏ *In-training　$88

Critical Care
❏ Individual　$165
❏ Institutions　$266
❏ *In-training　$83

Dental
❏ Individual　$150
❏ Institutions　$242

Emergency Medicine
❏ Individual　$170
❏ Institutions　$263
❏ *In-training　$85
　❏ Send CME info

Facial Plastic Surgery
❏ Individual　$199
❏ Institutions　$300

Foot and Ankle
Individual　$160
Institutions　$232

Gastroenterology
❏ Individual　$190
❏ Institutions　$276

Gastrointestinal Endoscopy
❏ Individual　$190
❏ Institutions　$276

Hand
❏ Individual　$205
❏ Institutions　$319

Heart Failure (NEW in 2005!)
❏ Individual　$99
❏ Institutions　$149
❏ *In-training　$49

Hematology/ Oncology
❏ Individual　$210
❏ Institutions　$315

Immunology & Allergy
❏ Individual　$165
❏ Institutions　$266

Infectious Disease
❏ Individual　$165
❏ Institutions　$272

Clinics in Liver Disease
❏ Individual　$165
❏ Institutions　$234

Medical
❏ Individual　$140
❏ Institutions　$244
❏ *In-training　$70
　❏ Send CME info

MRI
❏ Individual　$190
❏ Institutions　$290
❏ *In-training　$95
　❏ Send CME info

Neuroimaging
❏ Individual　$190
❏ Institutions　$290
❏ *In-training　$95
　❏ Send CME inf0

Neurologic
❏ Individual　$175
❏ Institutions　$275

Obstetrics & Gynecology
❏ Individual　$175
❏ Institutions　$288

Occupational and Environmental Medicine
❏ Individual　$120
❏ Institutions　$166
❏ *In-training　$60

Ophthalmology
❏ Individual　$190
❏ Institutions　$325

Oral & Maxillofacial Surgery
❏ Institutions　$180
❏ Institutions　$280
❏ *In-training　$90

Orthopedic
❏ Individual　$180
❏ Institutions　$295
❏ *In-training　$90

Otolaryngologic
❏ Individual　$199
❏ Institutions　$350

Pediatric
❏ Individual　$135
❏ Institutions　$246
❏ *In-training　$68
　❏ Send CME info

Perinatology
❏ Individual　$155
❏ Institutions　$237
❏ *In-training　$78
　❏ Send CME info

Plastic Surgery
❏ Individual　$245
❏ Institutions　$370

Podiatric Medicine & Surgery
❏ Individual　$170
❏ Institutions　$266

Primary Care
❏ Individual　$135
❏ Institutions　$223

Psychiatric
❏ Individual　$170
❏ Institutions　$288

Radiologic
❏ Individual　$220
❏ Institutions　$331
❏ *In-training　$110
　❏ Send CME info

Sports Medicine
❏ Individual　$180
❏ Institutions　$277

Surgical
❏ Individual　$190
❏ Institutions　$299
❏ *In-training　$95

Thoracic Surgery (formerly Chest Surgery)
❏ Individual　$175
❏ Institutions　$255
❏ *In-training　$88

Urologic
❏ Individual　$195
❏ Institutions　$307
❏ *In-training　$98
　❏ Send CME info

BUSINESS REPLY MAIL
FIRST-CLASS MAIL   PERMIT NO 7135   ORLANDO FL

POSTAGE WILL BE PAID BY ADDRESSEE

PERIODICALS ORDER FULFILLMENT DEPT
ELSEVIER
6277 SEA HARBOR DR
ORLANDO FL 32821-9816